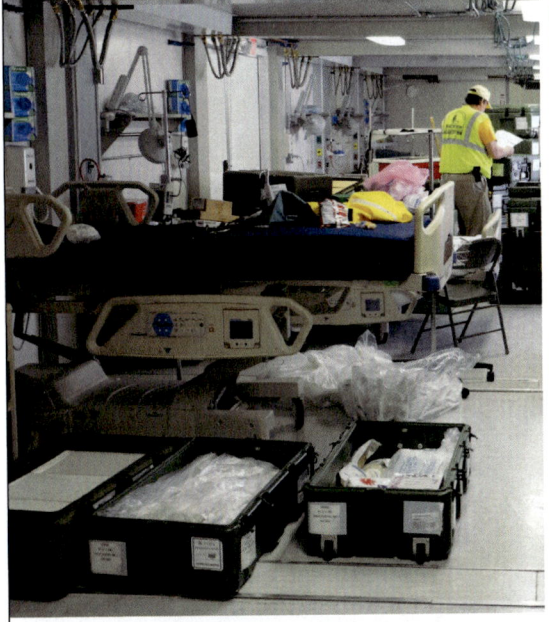
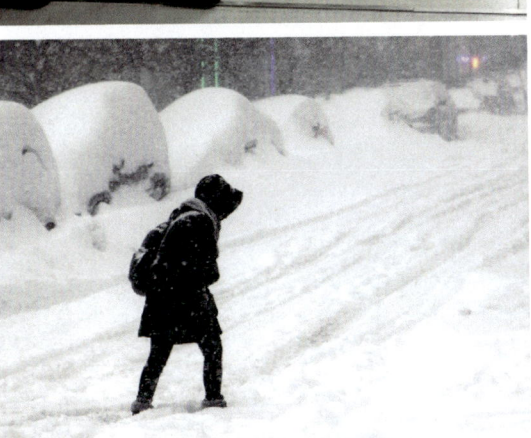
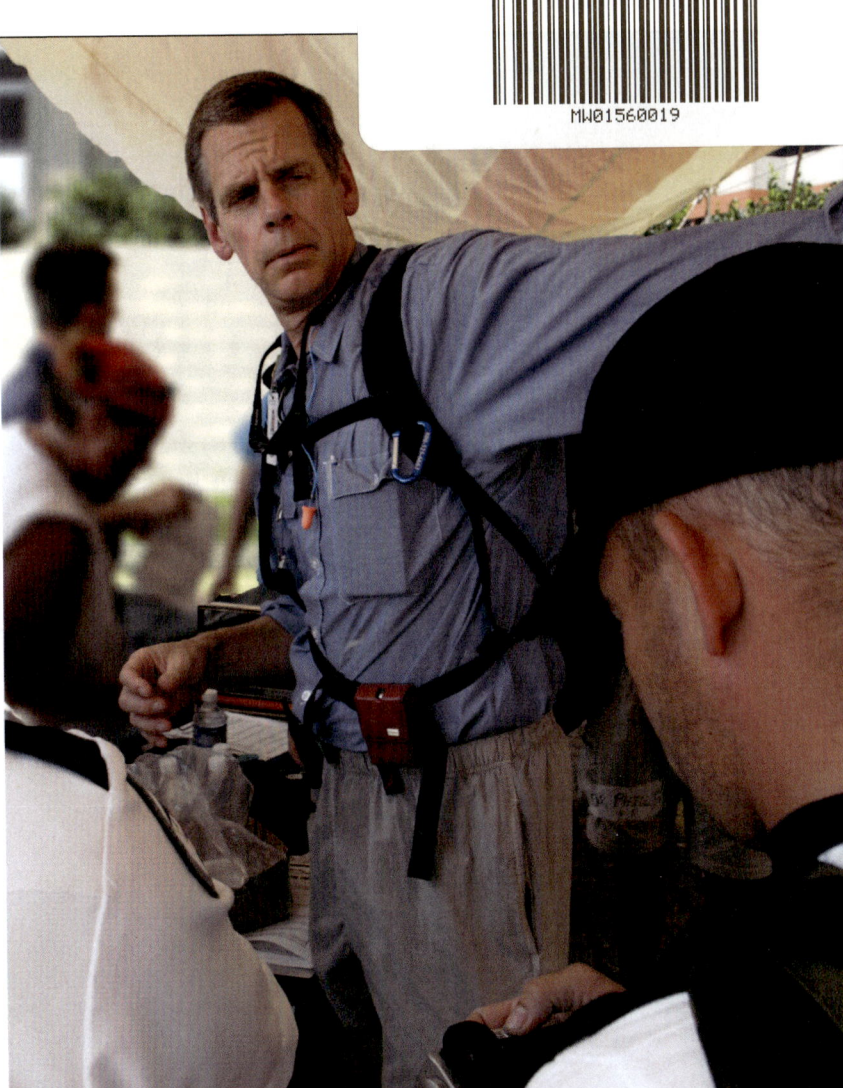

Emergency Management in Health Care
An All-Hazards Approach

THIRD EDITION

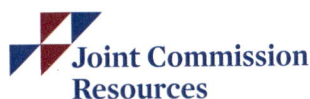

Joint Commission Resources

Foreword by
Ed Tangredi Jr., MS, CEM

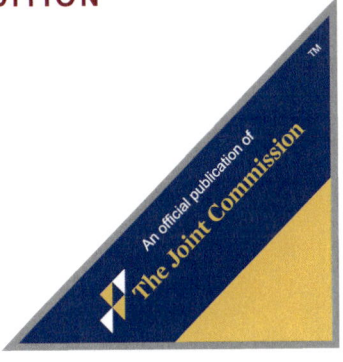

An official publication of The Joint Commission

Senior Editor: Laura Hible

Project Manager: Lisa King

Associate Director, Publications: Helen M. Fry, MA

Associate Director, Production and Meeting Support: Johanna Harris

Executive Director, Publications and Education: Catherine Chopp Hinckley, MA, PhD

Joint Commission and Joint Commission Resources Reviewers for the third edition: Lynne Bergero, John Maurer, Jim Kendig, Lisa Waldowski, Diane Sosovec, Doreen Finn, Jim Parker

External Reviewers: Ed Tangredi, Philip Niemer

Joint Commission Resources Mission

The mission of Joint Commission Resources (JCR) is to continuously improve the safety and quality of health care in the United States and in the international community through the provision of education, publications, consultation, and evaluation services.

Joint Commission Resources educational programs and publications support, but are separate from, the accreditation activities of The Joint Commission. Attendees at Joint Commission Resources educational programs and purchasers of Joint Commission Resources publications receive no special consideration or treatment in, or confidential information about, the accreditation process.

The inclusion of an organization name, product, or service in a Joint Commission Resources publication should not be construed as an endorsement of such organization, product, or service, nor is failure to include an organization name, product, or service to be construed as disapproval.

This publication is designed to provide accurate and authoritative information in regard to the subject matter covered. Every attempt has been made to ensure accuracy at the time of publication; however, please note that laws, regulations, and standards are subject to change. Please also note that some of the examples in this publication are specific to the laws and regulations of the locality of the facility. The information and examples in this publication are provided with the understanding that the publisher is not engaged in providing medical, legal, or other professional advice. If any such assistance is desired, the services of a competent professional person should be sought.

© 2016 The Joint Commission

Joint Commission Resources, Inc. (JCR), a not-for-profit affiliate of The Joint Commission, has been designated by The Joint Commission to publish publications and multimedia products. JCR reproduces and distributes these materials under license from The Joint Commission.

All rights reserved. No part of this publication may be reproduced in any form or by any means without written permission from the publisher.

Printed in the USA 5 4 3 2 1

Requests for permission to make copies of any part of this work should be mailed to
Permissions Editor
Department of Publications and Education
Joint Commission Resources
1515 W. 22nd Street, Suite 1300W
Oak Brook, Illinois 60523 USA
permissions@jcrinc.com

ISBN: 978-1-59940-937-5

Cover art: Photograph of Erik A. Larsen, MD, FACEP, taken by Michael Rieger for the Federal Emergency Management Agency. New Orleans, September 6, 2005. Courtesy of FEMA.

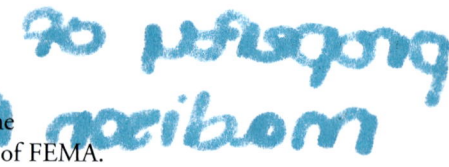

For more information about Joint Commission Resources, please visit http://www.jcrinc.com.

Table of Contents

Foreword vii

Introduction xi

CHAPTER 1: A Framework for Preparedness .1
Key Concepts for Emergency Management 1
    Figure 1-1. Possible Hazards. 2
Leadership's Role. 3
    Figure 1-2. Building a Team 4
The Four Phases of Emergency Management 4
The Six Critical Areas of Emergency Management. 6
Pulling Together the Right Players 8

CHAPTER 2: The Emergency Operations Plan 9
Key Concepts for the Emergency Operations Plan 10
    Figure 2-1. Process Steps for an Effective HVA 11
    Figure 2-2. Four Phases Code Chart. 12
    Figure 2-3. Sample Hazard Vulnerability Analysis 13
Case in Point Crozer-Keystone Health System Copes with the Security Measures Surrounding the Pope's Visit to Philadelphia 14
Best Practices for Success 18
Case in Point Extreme Weather Event: Hospitals in Baltimore and Clarksburg, West Virginia, Cope with Heavy Snowfall Blanketing the Area 19
    Figure 2-4. 96-Hour Operational Impact Chart. 23
    Figure 2-5. Incident Command Structure Leadership Responsibilities. 24
    Figure 2-6. Incident Commander. 26
Special Report 32

CHAPTER 3: Establishing and Facilitating Communications 37
Key Planning Concepts for Communications 37
    Figure 3-1. *Sample Communications List* 41
Case in Point Information Technology Outage at Yale New Haven Health 47
    Figure 3-2. *Incident Escalation for Disaster Declaration Review.* 48

CHAPTER 4: Managing Resources and Assets 55
Key Planning Concepts for Resources and Assets 55
    Figure 4-1. *Disaster Preparedness Budget.* 56

CHAPTER 5: Ensuring Safety and Security 65
Key Planning Concepts for Safety and Security 65
Case in Point Active Shooter Incident at Health First-Palm Bay Hospital. 67
Case in Point University of Maryland Medical Center in Baltimore Finds Itself
in the Middle of a Rioting City. 70

CHAPTER 6: Preparing Staff to Respond 79
Key Planning Concepts for Staff Response 80
Case in Point Effective Disaster Response Relies on First-Class EC Training for Staff . . . 82
    Figure 6-1. *Evaluation and Management of Patients.* 91
Case in Point Deadly EF5 Tornado Ravages Hospital and Requires Evacuation. 92
    Figure 6-2. *Granting Disaster Privileges and Assigning Disaster Responsibilities.* 96

CHAPTER 7: Safeguarding Utilities 97
Key Planning Concepts for Utilities 97
    Figure 7-1. *Emergency Power Preparation Checklist* 99
Case in Point Sutter Medical Center in Sacramento Responds
to a Loss of Backup Power 108

CHAPTER 8: Caring for Patients 111
Key Planning Concepts for Patient Care 111
    Figure 8-1. *Sample Shelter Triage Form.* 116
    Figure 8-2. *Sample Patient Tracking Form.* 123
    Figure 8-3. *Sample Patient Evacuation Tracking Form* 124
Case in Point A Hawaiian Hospital's Response to an Earthquake 126

CHAPTER 9: A Framework for Testing and Evaluation 129
Key Concepts for Testing and Evaluation 129
Case in Point Communitywide Emergency Response Exercise and Operating Room
   Evacuation Drill 134
   Figure 9-1. *Planning Matrix.* 136
   Figure 9-2. *Emergency Management: Exercise Planning Guide.* 138
Case in Point University of Nebraska Medical Center/Nebraska Medicine's
Biocontainment Unit Uses a Collaborative Model to Treat Patients Infected
with Ebola Virus Disease 139
   Figure 9-3. *Planning for Patients with Infectious Disease* 141
   Figure 9-4. *After-Action Review Sample* 143

CHAPTER 10: After the Incident 149
Key Concepts for Recovery 149
   Figure 10-1. *Downtime and Recovery Documentation Form.* 153
Case in Point Cape Canaveral Hospital Hit with Three Hurricanes in Seven Weeks 155
Case in Point Bon Secours Baltimore: Better than Before 158

Glossary 161

Index 165

Foreword

Like so many of you, when I started in the field of emergency preparedness I didn't know anything about its formal doctrine; all I knew was my life experience. The sudden tragedy of 9/11 transformed the worldview and scope of responsibilities for those of us in the field of emergency preparedness. More than ever, the impact of this event reinforced our commitment to the organizations we served. The Joint Commission provided us with standards and direction to keep our facilities safe during disasters and to equip staff with training to confront emergencies and save lives. We were given the task of writing an Emergency Operations Plan.

Over the years, The Joint Commission has established standards to ensure consistency across health care organizations and communicated the urgency of Emergency Management (EM) standards by assigning them their own chapter in The Joint Commission's accreditation manuals. This move truly signaled the importance of disaster preparedness and response in all health care organizations.

How far we have come! It has been a long journey for emergency managers—from minimal involvement of administration in planning processes and a lack of staff understanding of our roles. The concept of "exercise" no longer means time in the gym; instead it represents how we test the training and response of our staff and facility operations to a disaster. Full-time emergency managers learn to develop response plans for incidents such as infectious agents, active shooters, civil unrest, and even cyber attacks. Across our nation, health care organizations' Incident Command Structure staff have learned to manage crisis situations.

Of the many tools available to orient and train our staff throughout the organization, this third edition of *Emergency Management in Health Care: An All-Hazards Approach* provides a detailed and resourceful guide to navigating emergencies. As an emergency manager, I find, for example, the wealth of information on active shooter response and exercise design to be focused in a way that makes it useful. I used the previous edition to address two paramount areas of emergency preparedness when I wrote the "Code Silver: Active Shooter Response" plan and the "Ebola (Infectious Agent) Response" plan for my organization.

The six critical areas of emergency management focus all we do in emergency preparedness:
- Communications, the topic that comes up in every evaluation
- Resources and assets, supported by coalition building and mutual aid agreements
- Safety and security of staff, patients, and visitors
- Staff responsibilities, and support of staff and their families
- Utilities
- Patient clinical and support activities

Together, these all lay the groundwork for a program that is critical to our goal—life preservation, property protection, and incident stabilization. These are topics in the emergency preparedness world that never become second nature but do become possible with collaboration and resiliency.

The descriptions, examples, and tools included in this book make it possible to prepare for an active shooter, an emerging infectious disease patient, civil unrest in our community, ice storm, catastrophic flood, or a mass-casualty incident, all with a focus on crisis standards of care. At White Plains Hospital where I serve as director of Emergency Management, I have personally put these resources to work in developing our emergency preparedness plans and exercises. In collaboration with the White Plains Police Department, previous editions of *Emergency Management in Health Care: An All-Hazards Approach* have helped us to design, execute, and evaluate an active shooter exercise that participating staff described as some of the most intense moments of their careers. Along with the White Plains Fire Department, we have revised our evacuation plans and conducted exercises on blast injuries to all our community partners, with firsthand education provided by Dr. Erik Larsen, our associate director of the Emergency Department. Working with the Westchester County Department of Health, not only have we revised our infectious disease protocols, we have tested them when confronted with a possible smallpox patient.

Through the Hudson Valley MACE (Mutual Aid Coordinating Entity) team, a group of emergency managers whose hospitals—31 in total—are signatory to a mutual aid agreement, supporting each other in emergency preparedness efforts and exercises in the wake of declining Office of the Assistant Secretary for Preparedness and Response grant funding. We have come together in large and small events to support our partners. We have helped hospitals acquire instrument sterilization when they had a boiler fire and lost steam pressure. On another occasion we were able to get an incident hospital the staff and supplies they needed during Hurricane Sandy. Most recently the MACE team was the principle resource for patient placement at a National Disaster Medical System exercise. A military C-130 aircraft arrived, and as local emergency medical services (EMS) performed triage, the MACE team coordinated bed availability throughout the seven surrounding counties. This information was critical to timely patient disposition through the EMS Transportation Office.

Where am I going with all of the above examples? Coalitions! Successful emergency preparedness is truly about coalition building. Breaking down the barriers that separate health care, public safety, and community response has become the highest priority in emergency planning. When we build true coalitions, it all comes together in a way that enables the health care organization to provide a safe and secure health care environment at its highest levels. How do we do this? First we begin by inviting all key players to participate. In White Plains we have established an emergency preparedness task force that meets quarterly. At the table are public safety agencies such as the fire and police departments, county Office of Emergency Management (OEM), county Department of Health, state OEM, EMS, utility providers, and all the health care providers in the city.

Together we plan for known events, train for unknown events, and design and execute exercises. I speak often about our coalition successes, and they have become a unified command example for many other communities. Granted, it is not an easy task. Coalition building is one of the most complex challenges of my career. There are egos to check at the door, differences in style, and varied life experiences and perspectives. However, we all have the same drive and determination—our purpose for entering this field in the first place—quality patient care. We are all part of the same team, and protecting life and preventing injuries is the core mission of all we do. Joint Commission Resources provides the groundwork for meeting and exceeding that goal with this book, walking the reader through steps of designing, implementing, and executing a comprehensive emergency preparedness program.

I truly hope you find the resources and tools in this book helpful. I have and I continue to use it as a source when reviewing my own plans and procedures. It has become the go-to book for me when I need to get back to center, and it reminds me that all we do as emergency managers is based on an "all-hazards" approach.

Thank you for all you do in providing a safe and secure environment of care for our patients!

Ed Tangredi Jr., MS, CEM

Introduction

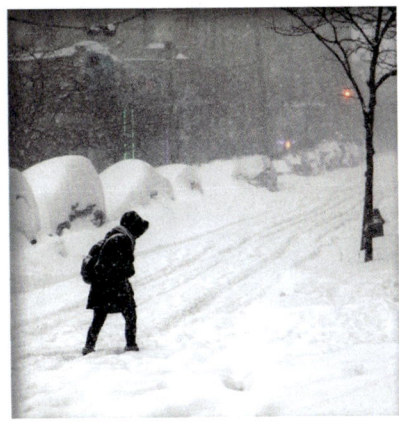

January 2016 heralded the arrival of Winter Storm Jonas, with its primary strike affecting a number of states in the eastern region of the country. Fortunately, its timing was not a surprise. The areas that would be hit the hardest had almost a week to prepare, receiving warnings and forecasts associated with the approaching storm several days in advance. Forecasters were predicting that many areas would receive between 10 and 18 inches of snow—the kind of snowfall that had the potential to cut hospitals and other health care organizations off from the community, from authorities, and even from their own staff.

Many of the health care organizations that stood in the path of the storm made early decisions to initiate their Emergency Operations Plan (EOP), alerting senior leadership and coordinating with local, state, and federal agencies to plan for food, pharmaceuticals, linens, and other supplies. As the storm drew near, staff were given to understand that they would likely be staying through the weekend because the roads would soon be impassable. Jonas dumped nearly 20 inches of snow over many areas in a day and a half.

Thorough planning, effective communication, and a coordinated response kept hospitals functioning relatively normally as Jonas raged outside. With a major storm whose impact had the potential to unleash widespread havoc, many health care organizations demonstrated how preparation and communication form the underpinnings of effective emergency response. The lessons learned there apply to all sorts of emergency situations from floods, to fires, to terrorist attacks and outbreaks of infectious disease. As Meg Femino, director of Emergency Management at Beth Israel Deaconess Medical Center in Boston, put it, "Hope is not a strategy." Effective emergency management—that is, maintaining the safety and security of staff and patients and continuing to fulfill the health care organization's mission—relies on planning, training, communication, superior organization, and strong, flexible leadership.

Goal of This Book

As domestic and global threats evolve, from weather-related events to infectious diseases to intensified terrorist attacks, it becomes ever more critical for health care organizations to engage in the kind of "all-hazards" emergency planning that will allow them to adapt on the fly to new and unanticipated threats and emergency situations. The goal of this book is to provide a comprehensive guide to emergency planning, mitigation, response, and recovery for organizations across the continuum of care.

Audience of This Book

Specifically, this book is intended for new emergency managers, either to health care or to the role or organization, and others involved in the multidisciplinary planning and application of the EOP, and new to their role in emergency preparedness—such as safety officers, facilities managers, medical and nursing directors, department heads, and clinical and support staff in all health care settings. Seasoned leaders in these roles will benefit from reading about the experiences of other health care organizations.

Purpose of This Book

This revision has six main goals:
1. To emphasize the role of leadership in emergency planning and response
2. To help organizations adapt to singular or escalating threats such as infectious disease outbreaks, acts of terrorism, active shooters, industrial accidents, unusual weather occurrences, and other emergencies
3. To expose the vulnerabilities that may impact technology in disaster responses—such as failures to manage resources, utilities, and systems processes
4. To identify technology advancements that may increase security in the use of electronic medical records
5. To update discussion of Joint Commission standards to reflect current requirements
6. To introduce the concept of continuity of operations (COOP) to health care emergency managers

Structure and Content of This Book

For ease of use, *Emergency Management in Health Care: An All-Hazards Approach,* 3rd Edition is broken into three sections.

Part 1—The Basics of Emergency Management Planning

This section covers the foundational concepts involved in emergency management, including interacting with key stakeholders, understanding key concepts, and developing an emergency operations plan.

Chapter 1: A Framework for Preparedness provides emergency planning and response.

Chapter 2: The Emergency Operations Plan walks the reader through the steps of assessing risk vulnerabilities and creating a comprehensive and adaptable EOP.

Part 2—Specific Areas of Response

Accreditation manuals for all settings—hospitals and critical access hospitals, home care, behavioral health care, ambulatory health care, and laboratories—have the "Emergency Management" (EM) chapter, and all settings have up to six critical areas that need to be protected for the organization to effectively respond to and recover from emergencies. This book covers the six critical areas of emergency management addressed by the Joint Commission standards. The chapters in this section include a description of the area's importance, the collaborative nature of planning in that particular area, and key planning concepts, as well as case studies, tools, charts, resources, and infographics.

Chapter 3: Establishing and Facilitating Communications

Chapter 4: Managing Resources and Assets

Chapter 5: Ensuring Safety and Security

Chapter 6: Preparing Staff to Respond

Chapter 7: Safeguarding Utilities

Chapter 8: Caring for Patients

Part 3—Testing the Plan and Preparing to Recover

This section covers the activities involved in planning emergency exercises, monitoring and evaluating responses to tests or actual emergencies, and planning for recovery and business continuity.

Chapter 9: A Framework for Testing and Evaluation provides information and tools for testing the EOP and keeping it up to date.

Chapter 10: After the Incident addresses issues involved in post-disaster recovery and COOP.

EMERGENCY MANAGEMENT IN HEALTH CARE: An All-Hazards Approach | Third Edition

Chapter Features

A number of new features in the third edition will help readers find and use the information that is most useful to them. These features are shown below.

Chapter Feature	Purpose
STANDARDS FOCUS	Identifies the concepts from the Joint Commission standards that are addressed in the chapter
AT A GLANCE	Details the main concepts addressed in each chapter
Why Is This Critical?	Explains the importance of each major concept addressed
WHO IS INVOLVED?	Lists personnel who may be involved in planning activities
 Community Collaboration	Highlights collaborative relationships and support structures for health care organizations
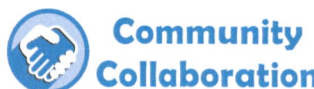 Setting Spotlight	Provides tools, tips, and resources for ambulatory health care, home care, nursing care centers, behavioral health care, and laboratory settings
Vulnerable Populations	Identifies populations requiring special consideration in planning activities
Capacity Builder	Provides additional resources, checklists, tools, and links that can help in emergency planning and preparedness
Threat Analysis	Identifies challenges to emergency preparedness concepts
IN SUMMARY	Summarizes the main concepts in the chapter
 Case in Point	Shares lessons learned and actions applied in case study organizations

Federal Rule

The Centers for Medicare & Medicaid Services (CMS) released in September 2016 its final rule for Emergency Preparedness Requirements for Medicare and Medicaid Participating Providers and Suppliers (*see* http://federalregister.gov/a/2016-21404). The Joint Commission Emergency Management standards referenced in this third edition of *Emergency Management in Health Care: An All-Hazards Approach* are comprehensive in their scope and hold accredited organizations to the most contemporary standards for planning and preparedness; CMS utilized these standards in developing the final rule. This book provides a comprehensive framework for health care organizations to prepare for the expanded federal rule for all-hazards planning, communications, exercises, and other requirements that build organization readiness and resilience. In particular, integrated systems and health care coalitions will find a wealth of examples and lessons learned for collaborating with response partners across settings and disciplines, supporting health care organizations in the movement from organization resilience to community resilience.

A Word About Terminology

Throughout this book, we use the term *Emergency Operations Plan (EOP)*. Ambulatory and behavioral health care organizations create an Emergency Management Plan (EMP) instead of an (EOP) but they're similar in intent. We also use the word *patient* to describe the care recipient, consumer, resident, individual receiving care, or the person who actually receives health care services.

Acknowledgments

We wish to express our appreciation to those members of the Joint Commission and Joint Commission Resources staff who reviewed the manuscript and/or advised in its development—especially Lynne Bergero, John Maurer, Jim Kendig, and Lisa Waldowski. We would also like to thank Philip Niemer, Children's Hospital Colorado, for his expert assistance and review. We extend our thanks to our Foreword writer, Ed Tangredi, White Plains Hospital, for his generosity and contributions to the manuscript.

In addition, we are grateful for the real-world scenarios provided by Grant Gegwich with Crozer-Keystone Health System, Carrie Russell with Highland Clarksburg Hospital, Karen Lancaster with the University of Maryland Medical Center, James Paturas with Yale New Haven Health, Jim Kendig for Health First, Mark Kaldahl with Carilion Franklin Memorial Hospital, Nancy Corbett with Mercy Health System, Nancy Turner with Sutter Medical Center, Michelle Schwedhelm with the University of Nebraska Medical Center/Nebraska Medicine, and Meg Femino with Beth Israel Deaconess Medical Center. Finally, we would like to thank our writer, James Foster, for his careful attention to detail and his consummate professionalism.

CHAPTER 1

A Framework for Preparedness

STANDARDS FOCUS

- **EM.01.01.01** The organization engages in planning activities prior to developing its written Emergency Operations Plan.
- **EM.02.01.01** The organization has an Emergency Operations Plan.
- **LD.04.01.05** The organization effectively manages its programs, services, sites, or departments.
- **LD.04.04.01** Leaders establish priorities for performance improvement.

AT A GLANCE

- Concepts in emergency planning
- Leadership in emergency management
- Teamwork to create an effective plan

DEFINING TERMS

emergency An unexpected or sudden event that significantly disrupts an organization's ability to provide care, or the environment of care itself; or that results in a sudden, significantly changed, or increased demand for the organization's services.

disaster A type of emergency that, due to its complexity, scope, or duration, threatens an organization's capabilities and requires outside assistance to sustain patient care, safety, or security functions.

emergency management The overarching discipline that ensures that organizations are building and testing plans utilizing the four phases of emergency management.

surge event Unexpected influx of patients that has the potential to or has overwhelmed organizational resources (for example, mass casualty, epidemic, flu).

Key Concepts for Emergency Management

From hurricanes, floods, and tornadoes, to transportation accidents and building collapses, to terrorist acts, mass shootings, and infectious disease outbreaks, the sheer variety of possible emergency situations means that organizations should take an "all-hazards" approach to emergency management (*see* Figure 1-1 on page 2). By building plans that are flexible and implementing incident command philosophies, organizations create a framework for emergency response. Regardless of the event, the overall impact of such situations can be reduced when health care organizations prepare staff, assess risks, develop and test contingency plans, and respond before a disaster hits.

The Joint Commission Emergency Management (EM) standards provide guidance to organization leaders to achieve this level of preparedness. After examining lessons learned from health care organizations impacted by large-scale disasters, The Joint Commission identified six critical areas of emergency response:

1. Communications
2. Resources and assets
3. Safety and security
4. Staff responsibilities
5. Utilities
6. Patient clinical and support activities

When organizations prepare and build resilience in each of these areas of emergency management, they have developed an "all-hazards" approach enabling them to address a wide range of emergencies.

The Emergency Operations Plan

Emergencies are a threat to any organization, regardless of size, scope, or location. A single emergency can temporarily affect demand for services, but escalating events—multiple emergencies that occur at the same time or occur one after another—can have even more serious consequences for patient safety and an organization's ability to provide care, treatment, and services for an extended length of time. This is particularly true in situations in which the community cannot adequately support the health care organization.

Figure 1-1. Possible Hazards

The list below is just a sample of the possible hazards to which health care organizations may need to respond. It is by no means exhaustive and does not include either disasters or events that may be caused or driven by more than one factor, or scenarios in which several of these events may happen simultaneously.

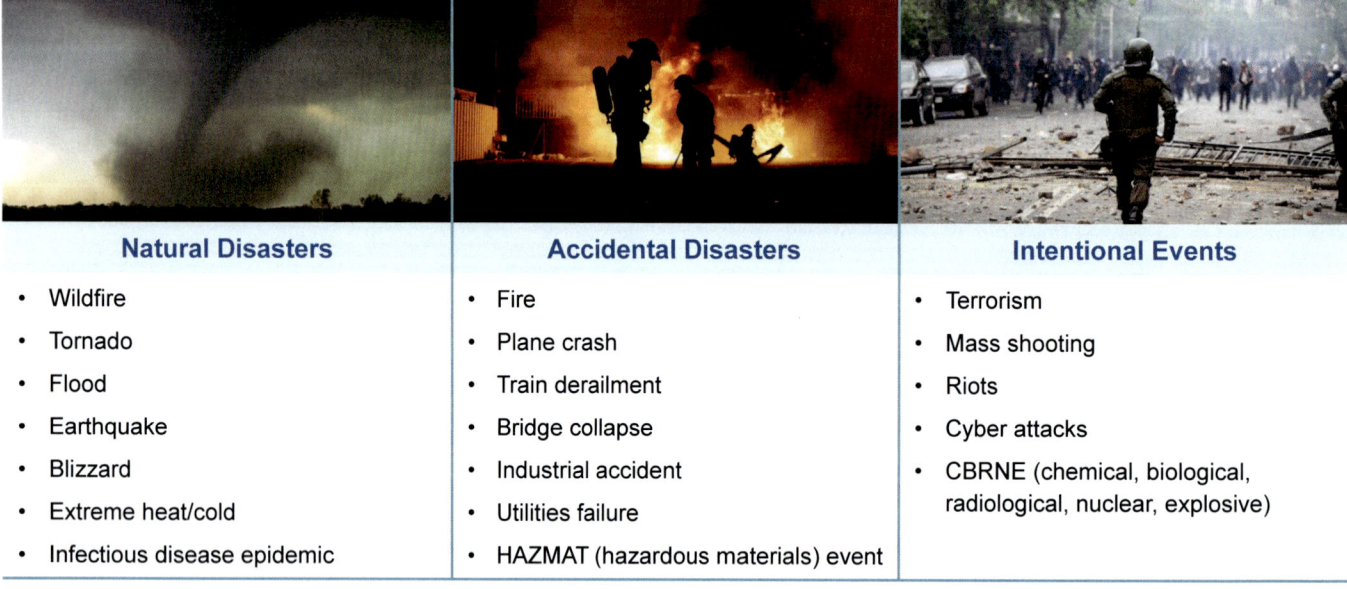

Natural Disasters	Accidental Disasters	Intentional Events
• Wildfire	• Fire	• Terrorism
• Tornado	• Plane crash	• Mass shooting
• Flood	• Train derailment	• Riots
• Earthquake	• Bridge collapse	• Cyber attacks
• Blizzard	• Industrial accident	• CBRNE (chemical, biological, radiological, nuclear, explosive)
• Extreme heat/cold	• Utilities failure	
• Infectious disease epidemic	• HAZMAT (hazardous materials) event	

Figure 1-1 presents various emergencies that organizations might encounter.

Power failures, water and fuel shortages, cyber attacks, loss of the EMR (electronic medical record), flooding, and communications breakdowns are just a few hazards that can disrupt care and pose risks to staff and the organization as a whole.

The Emergency Operations Plan (EOP)* is the organization's comprehensive plan for emergency and disaster response. Briefly, the EOP addresses all aspects of an organization's emergency operations across all six critical areas and moving through four phases of emergency management—mitigation, preparedness, response, and recovery. Chapter 2 will provide an in-depth discussion of the EOP's primary components.

The Hazard Vulnerability Analysis

Emergency planners begin developing an EOP by first preparing a hazard vulnerability analysis (HVA). The HVA is the fundamental tool for assessing hazards and risks to an organization's facilities and its ability to deliver services to the community. The HVA should be evaluated and updated by leaders on an annual basis and relevant information shared with community leaders. The process of creating the HVA, its evaluation and updating, and the prioritizing of the risks identified will be documented by members of the emergency management team. Chapter 2 will discuss the HVA in greater detail.

Leadership's Role

A successful emergency response depends on the involvement of organization leadership across all areas of the organization—operational, clinical, facilities, support, and so forth. The Joint Commission standards require leadership to participate in planning activities that lead to the development of the HVA. These activities include collaboration with community partners to understand both the risks in the community and potential support from the community that can mitigate risk. Leaders also confirm the role the organization will have in the community's incident command structure. They prioritize risks and make decisions regarding which mitigation and preparedness activities will be pursued, given the resources and role of the organization. A thorough review of the HVA guides the development of the written EOP. Senior leadership is responsible for assigning resources (through budgeting, staff assignment and training, facilities projects, procurement of equipment and supplies, and so forth) for preparedness across the organization, and supporting collaboration with coalition partners to build resilience. Leadership supports the incident command structure. Leadership is also responsible for participating in annual reviews of disaster planning and for reviewing any actual emergency responses in which the organization engages.

In addition, leaders will plan for recovery activities that will help the organization return to normal function as soon as possible after an emergency.

Leaders also will appoint an individual who is responsible for emergency management. This individual is ideally a full-time emergency manager; however, in many organizations, the person assigned to lead the emergency management functions also has additional responsibilities, typically as the facilities manager/engineer or safety/security manager.

---

* Depending on your health care setting, your organization may have an EOP or an Emergency Management Plan. For ease of discussion, we will use the term EOP inclusively for both concepts throughout this book.

Emergency Manager

The individual designated by leadership to lead emergency management will work with leaders across the organization and within the community to gather their input on vulnerabilities and gaps in preparedness (see Figure 1-2 below). Together, they will prepare a plan to address prioritized risk. He or she will oversee and facilitate emergency preparedness activities to enable cooperation across departments and foster a culture of teamwork. To do so, he or she must have access to resources and authority to make decisions regarding preparedness, mitigation, response, and recovery. He or she will be responsible for identifying and coordinating with outside entities, such as vendors, government agencies, community emergency response partners, and other health care organizations. Throughout the process, the emergency manager will coordinate all activities across the four primary phases of emergency management.

The Four Phases of Emergency Management

For each emergency prioritized in the HVA, organizations need to address four phases of emergency management: mitigation, preparedness, response, and recovery.

Figure 1-2. Building a Team

Emergency management planning should be a team process within the organization. A team approach brings increased creativity, knowledge, and experience to each phase of the emergency management planning process: mitigation, preparedness, response, and recovery.

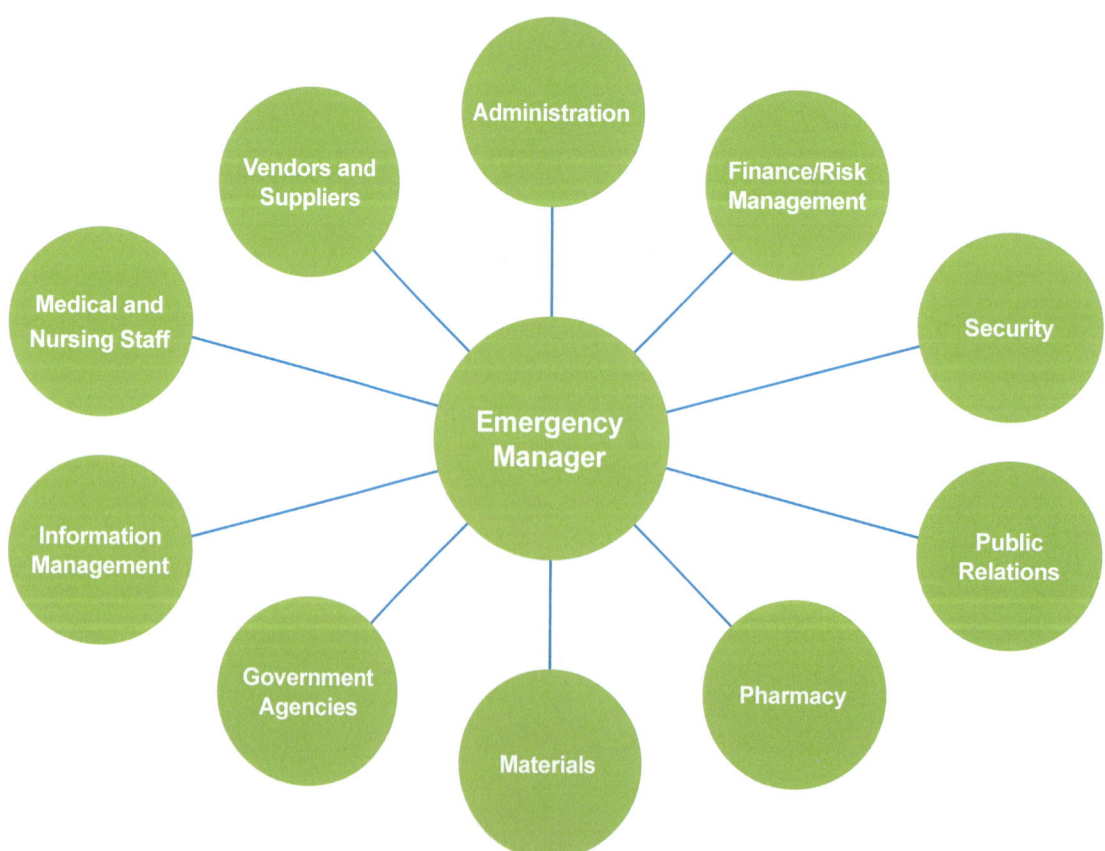

Figure 1-2 depicts departments and organizations that collaborate in emergency preparedness activities.

Mitigation

After the HVA identifies potential hazards, organizations can take steps to mitigate their vulnerability to certain kinds of emergencies. They might prepare utilities and other facilities to withstand disasters with little intervention. They might move information technology infrastructure off site to protect redundant capabilities. They might change security protocols to eliminate the opportunity for infant abductions. Finally, they need to establish alternative supply chains for food, water, medical supplies, fuel, and other essential provisions to prevent resource shortages.

Preparedness

Preparedness is the state of readiness that the organization has established to keep patients, staff, visitors, and facilities safe during an emergency. While the organization's EOP is generally a document, preparedness is the actual capability to respond using the staff, supplies, and space indicated in the EOP. For example, being prepared requires that the organization not only has described its intended response to pandemic flu, but that it has trained staff in patient surge management; acquired an initial inventory of essential medical and nonmedical supplies and established its supply chain for replenishing; developed and tested its triage plan with physicians, nurses, first responders, internal transport teams, unit staff, housekeeping, and other critical staff; and confirmed communication and coordination processes with public health and other authorities. Testing and exercising emergency response procedures are key components of preparedness. Regular emergency management exercises help organizations identify gaps in preparedness and help staff work together in agile teams in an evolving or escalating event. When staff participate in a simulation of a real-world situation, they will discover areas that need more attention. An evacuation drill, for example, might reveal failure to provide secure transfer of medical records, medications, and valuables. Identifying this kind of problem is the first step toward mitigating or correcting it.

Response

This is where all the planning comes into play. Leadership activates all or part of the organization's incident command structure according to the EOP so that the organization can continue to deliver essential services; manage resources; and protect patients, staff, and facilities. Depending on the type of emergency, response can range from managing a patient surge for 36 hours, to curtailing services to conserve resources, to a partial or full facility evacuation. A health care organization's response to an emergency strives to limit the effects on patient safety and care and reduce negative impact on staff and the facility.

Recovery

All emergencies end eventually. The organization defines the parameters for terminating emergency response and returning to normal operations. This can include repair of facilities; replenishing of supplies; updating of payroll, billing, and medical records; and the like. Depending on the emergency situation, staff may also need recovery time before returning to the usual routines and responsibilities of their jobs. Recovery also includes a thorough review of the event, an evaluation of the organization's response, and a plan to improve mitigation, preparedness, and response in the future.

Ensuring that operations continue during downtime is critical to meet the needs of patients, community, and staff. If the organization is unable to recover quickly from an unexpected event, serious patient harm or organizational damage, physical and reputational, may occur. Discussion on how a continuity of operations plan works with the Emergency Operations Plan is included in Chapter 10.

The Six Critical Areas of Emergency Management

The Joint Commission Emergency Management standards identify six areas of response that must be identified and considered as the organization's emergency management teams develop the EOP. These six areas are critical to the success of planning for and managing an emergency—regardless of its cause.

Communications

The receipt, review, and transmission of accurate and timely information is essential for situational awareness and coordination of response activities. Processes for communicating through the chain of command, with clinical and operational staff, patients, and response partners must be reliable and redundant. Any single communication pathway—e-mail, telephone (cellular, satellite, or landline), radio systems, Web-based programs, regional wireless communication networks, or other conduits—may fail in the event of an emergency. Outside factors could lead to the damage of community infrastructure and/or the debilitation of an organization's power or facilities. Organizations must develop a plan to maintain redundant communication pathways both within the organization and with critical community resources. Chapter 3 provides The Joint Commission's expectations related to communication.

Resources and Assets

A solid understanding of the availability of an organization's resources and assets is important in the evolving dynamics of an emergency or disaster. Materials and supplies, vendor and community services, as well as state and federal caches, are some of the essential resources that organizations must know how to access in times of crisis to help them maintain patient safety and sustain care, treatment, and services. Details regarding organizational planning for resources and assets during an emergency are located in Chapter 4.

Safety and Security

The safety and security of patients and staff is the prime responsibility of the organization during an emergency. Some safety strategies relate to damage of the health care facility due to natural or manmade events; in other situations the facility is intact but must be protected from unauthorized access, vandalism, or theft. In all cases, the secure access and movement of staff, patients, and visitors is paramount. Chapter 5 explores this plan component more thoroughly.

Staff Responsibilities

The emergency management standards address staff responsibilities, which can change during the course of an emergency. As conditions evolve and new risks emerge, staff will need to adapt their roles to meet new challenges to their abilities to care for patients. If staff cannot anticipate how they might be called on to perform during an emergency, the likelihood increases that the organization will not sustain itself during an emergency. Chapter 6 addresses issues associated with defining and managing staff roles and responsibilities during an emergency.

Capacity Builder

Besides Joint Commission standards, various aspects of emergency preparedness and response are governed by law and regulation. Below is a list of resources where emergency planners can find relevant legal and regulatory information.

FEMA and ASPR
The Federal Emergency Management Agency (FEMA) and Assistant Secretary for Preparedness and Response (ASPR) guidelines and requirements define the role organizations play in larger emergency response plans, including the National Incident Management System (NIMS) and the National Response Framework (NRF). Information on NIMS can be found online at http://www.fema.gov/national-incident-management-system and on NRF at https://www.fema.gov/media-library/assets/documents/32230.

OSHA
The Occupational Health and Safety Administration (OSHA) provides information on emergency planning in the context of worker safety and health at https://www.osha.gov/SLTC/emergencypreparedness/index.html.

NFPA
The National Fire Protection Association (NFPA) issues fire safety codes that pertain to health care facilities and emergency management. Relevant information can be found here:
Health Care Facilities Code: http://www.nfpa.org/codes-and-standards/nfpa-resources-for-cms-requirements-on-nfpa-99-and-nfpa-101

Disaster/Emergency Management Code: http://www.nfpa.org/codes-and-standards/document-information-pages?mode=code&code=1600

State and Local Laws and Regulations
Emergency planners can check with state and local public health and emergency management authorities for information on applicable laws and regulations.

CMS
The Centers for Medicare & Medicaid Services (CMS) has information on emergency preparedness, including checklists and tools for hospitals and long term care facilities here:
https://www.cms.gov/Medicare/Provider-Enrollment-and-Certification/SurveyCertEmergPrep/HealthCareProviderGuidance.html

CMS quarterly provider updates can be found here:
https://www.cms.gov/Regulations-and-Guidance/Regulations-and-Policies/QuarterlyProviderUpdates/index.html

The Joint Commission
The Joint Commission's Emergency Management Portal is dedicated to providing numerous emergency management resources:
http://www.jointcommission.org/emergency_management.aspx

Utilities

An organization depends on the uninterrupted function of its utilities during an emergency. Key utilities, such as power, potable water, ventilation, medical gases, and fuel, must be protected, and alternative sources for essential utilities must be established in advance. Discussion surrounding this requirement and the framework for managing this critical function appear in Chapter 7.

Patient Clinical and Support Activities

The clinical needs of patients during an emergency are of prime importance. The organization must have clear, reasonable plans to address the needs of patients during extreme conditions when the organization's infrastructure and resources are taxed. Chapter 8 examines the accreditation requirements related to managing patients and the clinical and support activities associated with them.

Pulling Together the Right Players

Emergency preparedness is a huge ongoing undertaking, and as such requires an organizationwide commitment. Medical staff will be the ones on the front lines of emergency response, so the perspective and experiences of medical staff leaders are invaluable resources when planning and preparing.

For example, in the case of a potential outbreak of infectious disease, the expertise of medical staff is essential to planning procedures for intake, housing, and care of infected patients. Given how resource- and labor-intensive the response may be to even a single patient with a highly infectious disease such as Ebola, it is easy to see why collaboration is critical to every phase of the planning process in all six areas of emergency management. Medical staff and support staff—including those responsible for the decontamination and disposal of materials used by infected patients—need to work together to provide for the safety of all people in the organization. An effective team includes staff from all areas of the organization, as well as internal and external vendors and suppliers, and community partners such as the health department, emergency management office, other governmental entities, and communications networks. Chapter 2 provides a more in-depth discussion of this partnership effort.

IN SUMMARY

- An all-hazards approach to emergency preparedness involves conducting a thorough HVA that leads to the creation of an EOP that covers all six critical areas of response across all four phases of emergency management.

- Organizational leaders are involved throughout the process, appointing the emergency manager, making decisions about planning and mitigation, directing reviews of planning and response, and helping to facilitate cooperation and implementation across departments.

- The emergency manager will oversee and facilitate implementation and cooperation, as well as identify and coordinate with outside agencies and partners.

CHAPTER 2

The Emergency Operations Plan

STANDARDS FOCUS

- **EM.01.01.01** The organization engages in planning activities prior to developing its written Emergency Operations Plan.
- **EM.02.01.01** The organization has an Emergency Operations Plan.
- **LD.04.01.05** The organization effectively manages its programs, services, sites, or departments.
- **LD.04.04.01** Leaders establish priorities for performance improvement.

AT A GLANCE

- Conducting the hazard vulnerability analysis
- Creating and maintaining the Emergency Operations Plan
- Working with collaboration partners
- Identifying the incident command structure
- Understanding crisis standards of care

Why Is This Critical?

The Emergency Operations Plan (EOP) lays the groundwork for every aspect of emergency management. An emergency, by definition, creates a substantial change or increase in demand for health care services. This means that emergency situations require hospital and health care organization leaders to make decisions amid extraordinary circumstances not covered under normal operations. An organization may be required to accommodate a surge in patients from a mass-casualty event or due to the evacuation of another health care facility nearby. Supply or utility disruptions may occur as a result of natural disasters, accidents, or civil unrest. The presentation of one or more potential infectious disease patients may necessitate a facility to initiate special triage, biocontainment, and infection control procedures.

To properly manage emergency situations, organizations need to identify and plan in advance for the most likely scenarios, while leaving enough flexibility in the plan to allow the emergency management team to respond to the unexpected. A hospital with a trauma unit located in an area with a lot of heavy industry should be prepared to manage a mass-casualty industrial accident. However, plans for such an event can be adapted to other kinds of mass-casualty events or patient surges, for instance. Sometimes multiple emergency situations coincide. For example, the staff of the Nebraska Biocontainment Unit, at the University Nebraska Medical Center, had to deal with a tornado warning during activation for treatment of patients with Ebola. Strong and flexible emergency planning is the best defense against the unexpected.

WHO IS INVOLVED?

- Organization administrative leadership
- Emergency manager
- Clinical staff leaders
- Community disaster response partners
- Vendors and suppliers
- Safety officer
- Facilities management

Key Concepts for the Emergency Operations Plan

What follows is a discussion of the key concepts in emergency management planning. Each organization will need to determine its vulnerabilities across its environment of care, prioritize risks, create a plan to mitigate or prepare to respond to threats, and create a comprehensive plan that takes into account its capabilities and is integrated into the larger organizational and community emergency response system.

Hazard Vulnerability Analysis

The process begins with organization leaders reviewing the Joint Commission Emergency Management (EM) standards to make sure they understand the requirements. They can then examine the functions of their organization affected by the standards and look for the most effective ways to meet the standards. The first step in addressing the emergency management standards is to perform a hazard vulnerability analysis (HVA). This analysis will provide a thorough evaluation of the organization's risks, the hazards it is likely to face, and the prioritizing of hazards. (*See* Figure 2-1 on page 11 for direction on beginning this process.) Leaders will use the findings of the HVA to determine the organization's ability to allocate resources, space and staff, and identify gaps in preparedness that need to be addressed. (*See* Figure 2-2 on page 12.) This process will provide the groundwork for the development of the EOP—a robust preparation for the most likely emergency scenarios.

Identify Hazards

Operational, clinical, and administrative leaders, and other staff, should gather to brainstorm a list of likely hazards to organization operations, including, but not limited to, naturally occurring, human-related, technological, utility-related, geographic, and other events, including terrorism. Staff should also consider events internal to the organization that may affect the delivery of services and care, such as loss of electricity service or fires. (*See* Figure 1-1 in the previous chapter.) Larger systems should consider conducting multiple HVAs, as the events based on location, services provided, and community resources may vary significantly.

Identifying hazards also involves working with external partners, such as health departments, fire departments, public works, police, and local and regional emergency response agencies, to help identify likely emergency scenarios. Some hazards may be related to geography (for instance, proximity to chemical plants or transit hubs). Likewise, the range of likely natural disasters is different depending on where the facility is located. A long term care facility in Arizona may want to pay special attention to the possibility of loss of air-conditioning in the summer, whereas a surgery center in Florida will need to plan extensively for hurricanes. Hazard analysis may be at the local or regional level.

Prioritize Risks

Next, leaders should prioritize hazards according to their potential likelihood and severity with respect to organization operations. Development of the EOP should be driven by the need to mitigate the effects of, prepare for, respond to, and recover from those events deemed most likely to occur and most likely to cause a major disruption in normal organization activities.

Figure 2-1. Process Steps for an Effective HVA

Developing and Maintaining an Effective HVA

An effective HVA doesn't just happen. Here are some suggested steps to help you develop one:

- ▶ **Step 1—Gather the team:** Host a brainstorming session with organization experts and representatives.
- ▶ **Step 2—Generate a list:** List potential emergencies. Make sure they're realistic for your region.
- ▶ **Step 3—Review historical data:** Look at information on emergencies over the past few decades in your region. Move to the top of the list any emergencies that have occurred previously in the community and/or the health care organization.
- ▶ **Step 4—Determine probability of occurrence:** For each type of emergency, determine the probability of occurrence. Make adjustments to the list order based on likelihood of occurrence.
- ▶ **Step 5—Assess impact:** Assess how each emergency would affect the organization and reorder accordingly.
  - If lives could be lost and safety is threatened, the emergency should move up on the list.
  - Evaluate the long-term effects of each emergency as well. For example, an influx of contaminated patients might require taking the emergency department (ED) offline for a long period of time.
  - Consider also how the organization's reputation could be damaged by a lack of preparedness.
- ▶ **Step 6—Conduct a gap analysis:** To determine emergencies that you aren't prepared for and the steps to fix that. Conduct a gap analysis.
- ▶ **Step 7—Do a community review:** Review the HVA with other emergency response agencies and health care organizations in the community to ensure compatibility.
- ▶ **Step 8—Participate in community preparedness:** To test your strategies, participate in community planning and emergency training activities.
- ▶ **Step 9—Review annually:** Review the HVA annually as a team.

Figure 2-1 shows process steps in developing the hazard vulnerability analysis (HVA).

An organization can develop its HVA by classifying hazards and placing them on a grid format. Hazards can be ranked by using a numbering system, such as the following:

1 = could occur or high likelihood
2 = might occur or moderate likelihood
3 = could never occur or no likelihood

The severity of the impact on the organization can be rated by using a high-, moderate-, low-, or no-impact ranking. Input from frontline staff from a variety of support areas—transportation, housekeeping, security, and so forth—will help surface logistical issues that can aid in rating severity of impact. Then the ranked hazards and impacts can be linked with the organization's resources that could be affected. Identifying how each resource will be affected by each hazard makes it possible for the organization to plan its response for potential emergencies. (*See* Figure 2-3 on page 13 for a sample HVA planning tool.)

The HVA should be reevaluated at least annually and updated as necessary using data and experience from emergency response exercises and any actual emergency responses conducted since the previous review in the community or state. A challenge with conducting annual evaluations is that most community partners do not use the same HVA tool or define the

Figure 2-2. Four Phases Code Chart

Event	Mitigation	Preparedness	Response	Recovery
Workplace Violence	• Security Procedures • Panic Buttons • Interaction with Outside Agencies • Facility Design • Staff Training • Risk Assessments • Patient/Visitor Assessment • Checklists • Photo IDs • Authorized Personnel Only Signs • Crisis Intervention Training	• Security Procedures • Security Plans • Discussion with Police • Staff Education • Coordination with Police and Fire Departments • Other Plans (e.g., Evacuation) • Workplace Violence Policy • Threat Assessment Team • Crisis Communication Plan	• Overhead Announcement • Implementation of Plan • Staff Response to Area • Security Access Control • Notification of Police • Security Procedures • Evacuation of Affected Area • Security Procedures • Search of Areas • Interview of Witnesses • Police Department Backup	• Records and Documentation • Debriefing and AAR Documentation • Critical Incident Stress Debriefing • Incident Reports • Facility Damage Reports • Financial Impact Analysis • Insurance Contacts

Figure 2-2 provides some of the top safety and security concerns that organizations might face in planning for a workplace violence event.

Source: Niemer P. Children's Hospital Colorado. Aurora, CO. Used with permission.

events similarly. Working with community partners to standardize tools, processes, and events prior to the evaluation will help to ensure a successful evaluation.

Evaluate Top Risks

After the top organizational risks have been identified, the emergency manager—with the support of leadership—should conduct a gap analysis to identify the activities already implemented. The analysis provides a clear picture of how the four phases are being impacted. Working with other internal and external partners may provide ideas not listed that the organization could consider implementing.

Figure 2-3. Sample Hazard Vulnerability Analysis

Event	PROBABILITY	SEVERITY = (MAGNITUDE − MITIGATION)					RISK
	Likelihood this will occur	Human Impact Possibility of death or injury	Property Impact Physical losses and damages	Business Impact Interruption of services	Preparedness Preplanning	Internal Response Time, effectiveness, resources	External Response Community/Mutual Aid staff and supplies	Relative threat*
Score	0 = N/A 1 = Low 2 = Moderate 3 = High	0 = N/A 1 = Low 2 = Moderate 3 = High	0 = N/A 1 = Low 2 = Moderate 3 = High	0 = N/A 1 = Low 2 = Moderate 3 = High	0 = N/A 1 = Low 2 = Moderate 3 = High	0 = N/A 1 = Low 2 = Moderate 3 = High	0 = N/A 1 = Low 2 = Moderate 3 = High	0–100%
Blizzard	0	3	3	3	0	0	0	0%
Dam Inundation	3	2	3	3	1	1	1	61%
Drought	3	3	2	2	2	1	2	67%
Earthquake	3	2	1	2	2	1	2	56%
Epidemic	2	3	2	3	1	1	1	41%
Flood, External	2	2	2	3	2	2	2	48%
Hurricane	1	1	2	2	2	2	2	20%
Ice Storm	0	2	3	3	0	0	0	0%
Landslide	2	2	0	1	3	3	1	37%
Severe Thunderstorm	2	1	0	1	3	3	2	37%
Snowfall	1	2	3	2	3	3	3	30%
Temperature Extremes	2	1	2	2	2	2	3	44%
Tidal Wave	1	2	2	2	3	3	3	28%
Tornado	0	0	2	2	3	3	3	0%
Volcano	0	0	3	3	0	0	0	0%
Wildfire	3	3	0	2	1	1	1	44%
Average Score	1.56	1.81	1.88	2.25	1.75	1.63	1.63	32%

RISK = PROBABILITY x SEVERITY		
0.32	0.52	0.61

Figure 2-3 is a sample HVA tool organizations might use.
Source: Kaiser Permanente, Oakland, CA. Used with permission.

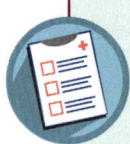

Case in Point
Crozer-Keystone Health System Copes with the Security Measures Surrounding the Pope's Visit to Philadelphia

A Preplanned Emergency

Preparations for the September 2015 visit of Pope Francis to Philadelphia began nearly six months prior to the event, as agencies from the US Secret Service and the Department of Homeland Security to the Pennsylvania Department of Health began to put together a plan to secure the safety of the pope and the hundreds of thousands of people who were expected to converge on the Center City district of Philadelphia at the end of September.

Emergency planners at Crozer-Keystone Health, which operates a network of five hospitals and numerous outpatient centers located primarily in neighboring Delaware County, knew the potential impact on its system could be substantial. The pope's visit was projected to entail the largest individual security operation in US history. So the staff at Crozer-Keystone used the months of advance warning to plan their response.

A Comprehensive Plan

The massive security operation next door presented a number of challenges to the organization. A large section of central Philadelphia would be fenced off, complicating access to several hospitals within the secure zone. Accordingly, Crozer-Keystone officials planned for a potential increase in patient load. The system includes a Level 2 trauma center and a regional burn center, so emergency planners had to plan for a patient surge that might stem from a mass-casualty event such as a terrorist attack or a transit accident. There was also the twofold challenge of limited mobility caused by a massive influx of people and the security measures meant to handle them. The bridges into Philadelphia would be closed. Major arterial streets would be closed for the duration of the pope's two-day visit. And the entire center of the city would be locked down. The mobility problems meant that some staff might have difficulty getting to work, patients might have difficulty getting to hospitals, and ambulance service might be adversely affected. Given that Crozer-Keystone is the largest provider of 911 services in Delaware County, this last challenge was of special concern.

The fact that hundreds of thousands of people would essentially be funneled into the public transportation system also increased the risk of a transit accident. With Amtrak and SEPTA commuter rail lines in close proximity to the network's facilities, the possibility of a mass-casualty transit accident had to be planned for as well.

Crozer-Keystone's emergency planning team took an analytical approach to the situation, breaking the complex situation down into smaller parts and forming subcommittees to tackle each facet of the problem. Committees were formed to focus on nursing issues, supplies, facilities, and so on. Preparations were made to house any staff who would be forced to stay at work over the weekend. As a precaution, patients scheduled to deliver babies that weekend and those at the top of the organ transplant lists were brought into the appropriate hospitals before the pope's arrival to ensure that they would not be prevented from reaching the hospital over the weekend. Planners worked with emergency medical services (EMS) to develop contingency plans for transporting patients during the high traffic period. Emergency departments and the trauma and burn centers were prepared to receive large numbers of patients. Extra supplies were obtained and organized, including self-sufficiency supplies to deal with supply disruptions.

The Event
Crozer-Keystone officials decided to coordinate their emergency management efforts from their organization's central incident command center. The incident command center was opened and the EOP was initiated at noon on Friday, September 25, the day before the papal visit. From noon Friday until noon Monday officials at the incident command center kept abreast of developments via the Pennsylvania Department of Health's Knowledge Center, a Web-based emergency management dashboard. The Knowledge Center allowed them to monitor security and emergency services alerts, as well as giving and receiving updated information such as bed censuses every two hours.

Emergency Operations Plan

With likely hazards identified and prioritized in the HVA, the organization must create the processes necessary to offer safe, high-quality care for patients in the face of an emergency. Joint Commission standards spell out the requirements for an all-hazards EOP. Following is a list of what the EOP must do at a basic level as identified by The Joint Commission:

- Describe mitigation activities
- Establish response procedures
- Assign roles and responsibilities
- Identify organization capabilities
- Collaborate with the community
- Determine alternative care sites
- Identify essential resources
- Describe recovery strategies

Describe Mitigation Activities

Like the EOP itself, mitigation begins with the HVA. After the planning team identifies and prioritizes risks to emergency preparedness, it can create a list of appropriate mitigation activities according to a multifactorial approach including a cost-benefit analysis. Each event may also be evaluated based on location, available resources, and culture. *Mitigation activities* are those actions an organization can take in advance of an emergency to reduce its vulnerability or to reduce the probable effects of certain kinds of emergencies. Leadership can assess how best to address mitigation. For instance, to reduce the vulnerability of an emergency department (ED) to active shooters or other violent actors, leaders might consider a number of options ranging from changing policies regarding visitor movement and access, to training ED personnel in de-escalation techniques and/or self-defense, to changes in security staffing and equipment, to enhancements to the building and security system. Every facility is different, and it is up to leaders and emergency planners to assess their facilities' particular risks and how best to allocate the organization's finite resources to manage them.

Establish Response Procedures

The planning team must develop organizationwide emergency response procedures that address the six critical areas described in Chapter 1: communications, resources and assets, safety and security, staff responsibilities, utilities, and patient clinical and support activities. Emergency response activities allow the organization to deal with the initial effects of an emergency; mitigate its effects on patients, staff, and the facility as it evolves; and support resilient recovery. Response procedures could include the following: maintaining or expanding services, conserving resources, curtailing services, supplementing resources from outside the local community, closing the organization to new patients, staged evacuation, and total evacuation.

Assign Roles and Responsibilities

To prevent confusion, the EOP must identify explicitly the person or persons with authority to initiate and terminate the response and recovery phases of the plan. The EOP must include an incident command structure (ICS) clarifying staff responsibilities and identifying the individuals who will make organizationwide decisions during an emergency, such as ordering an evacuation, speaking to the media or government organizations, and performing other executive functions. The ICS is critical to situational awareness, efficient decision making, and effective communication in chaotic or rapidly changing circumstances. The ICS will be discussed later in this chapter.

Identify Organization Capabilities

In the event of an emergency affecting the surrounding community, health care organizations must work together with government and community partners, as well as other health care organizations—some of which may at other times be competitors. Working as part of this broader disaster response framework, an organization must identify its emergency response capabilities. This includes such considerations as its ability to accommodate special needs populations, handle a patient surge, or house infectious disease patients. Special facilities such as burn centers, respiratory or other disease treatment centers, trauma centers, and neonatal resources should be incorporated into planning, training, and exercises. Special capabilities may also take the form of membership in regional or national coalitions with relevant specialties, such as treatment of traumatic injuries, burns, radiation exposure, or other conditions. A thorough and documented bed census and inventory of equipment is essential at the start of an incident and requires updating throughout response and recovery. Organizations should also evaluate the capability to manage pet care, elder care, and child care to ensure that staff are able to come to work.

Collaborate with the Community

Community collaboration is essential for comprehensive emergency management planning, and for resilient health care response and recovery. Community collaboration takes place through health care organizations reaching out to other health care providers, and to public health, public works, and public safety agencies, concerning areas of common interest. In recent years, such collaboration has proven effective in addressing many health care issues, resulting in increased support for health care coalitions to enhance disaster preparedness in communities. *A health care coalition* can be defined as a collaborative network of health care organizations and their respective public- and private-sector response partners that serve as a multiagency coordinating group to assist with mitigation, preparedness, response, and recovery activities related to health care organization disaster operations.[1] Health care coalitions facilitate resource sharing and staff training, enhance situational awareness during disasters, and extend the manpower pool for prolonged response and recovery. Health care coalitions can help smaller organizations (for example, home care, ambulatory, and behavioral health care providers) participate more effectively in emergency planning, training, and exercises. Increasing the number and type of health care providers prepared and available helps to increase the number of patients who can be cared for in the community.

Hurricanes, earthquakes, pandemic disease outbreaks, and other potential mass-casualty events will make it impossible for hospitals to serve the needs of all patients. Health care partners in the community are already serving patients who may be able to continue receiving care in the community during an emergency, leaving hospital beds available to care for only the most severely ill or injured. Including home care and ambulatory providers in planning up front helps to identify and locate vulnerable patients and proactively plan for the best location for their care during an emergency, be that in an inpatient or community-based setting.

Determine Alternative Care Sites

In the event of an evacuation or a patient surge that overwhelms organization capacity, staff and other responders must have plans in place to relocate patients to other health care facilities or approved alternative care sites. It is critical to identify potential alternative care sites ahead of time and establish relationships with the owners and operators of those sites. Failure to preplan may result in multiple community partners claiming the same alternate care location. During an emergency, such preexisting relationships can activate agreed-upon processes to facilitate proper placement of patients, staff, and equipment should evacuation be required. Emergency planners must think creatively about possible relocations sites (*see* the "Community Collaboration" sidebar on this page).

There is another important benefit to identifying and bringing to the table all the health care assets available in a community. When all partners are at the table—hospitals, home care, durable medical equipment, ambulatory surgery centers, outpatient dialysis providers, respiratory therapists, social workers, clinical psychologists, laboratory services, and so forth across the continuum of care—the expertise and skills they bring to patient care during a widespread disaster will enhance resilience and will help the community delay the moment it will have to activate a crisis standards of care response. *See* the "Special Report" section addressing crisis standards of care at the end of this chapter.

Identify Essential Resources

Organizations must conduct and maintain a thorough, documented inventory of resources essential for emergency response. Emergency conditions may interrupt the organization's supplies of medications, personal protective equipment, water (both potable and nonpotable), food, fuel, and so on. Organizations must ensure that they have on hand or have access to all essential resources in the event of an emergency.

Joint Commission standards require a hospital to monitor and manage its resources and assets during an emergency to project whether it can safely sustain patient care services for at least 96 hours. The hospital is not required to maintain a 96-hour inventory—it is required to project whether it can sustain services safely for at least 96 hours before it can be resupplied by the community (*see* Figure 2-4). This chapter addresses the 96-hour requirement in more length in a later section.

Community Collaboration

The following is a partial, non-exhaustive list of nontraditional sites in the community that may serve in an emergency as alternative care sites, evacuation centers, discharge or intake locations, or other needed functions.

- Aircraft hangars
- Closed hospitals or long term care facilities
- College dormitories
- Community/recreation centers
- Fairgrounds
- Government buildings
- Hotels/motels
- Libraries
- Meeting halls
- Military facilities
- National Guard armories
- Places of worship
- Schools
- Sports stadiums/facilities
- Tents
- Trailers
- Unleased/empty open-space buildings (such as grocery stores)
- Warehouses

Describe Recovery Strategies

After an emergency situation subsides, organizations need to return to normal operations as quickly as possible. Having business impact analysis and downtime/recovery plans in place beforehand is a critical step in efficiently returning to serving the community through the organization's core mission. It also provides strategies for those suffering long-term effects from the emergency. Recovery activities may include repair to facilities, updating of records, replenishing supplies, and other activities that return the organization to its pre-emergency footing. However, recovery will also include the evaluation of the organization's response and the possible development of recommendations to improve on that response in the future. Chapter 10 includes additional discussion on recovery.

Best Practices for Success

The Emergency Management standards require organizations to take a holistic approach to managing an emergency—not only preparing for a coordinated response but anticipating problems and ensuring self-sufficiency. Effective emergency management requires planning and preparation efforts and complete and total support from everyone in an organization—from leadership to frontline staff. Working with the community and other health care organizations, strengthening relationships with suppliers, and preparing for evacuations are key areas to consider when developing or improving an EOP.

Working with the Community

Emergency management planning should be done in the context of the community. An organization should know where it fits into a community response, including what services the organization can provide and what help and mutual aid can be expected.

Organizations should coordinate with local community emergency responders (such as the police department, the fire department, and emergency medical technicians), the local public health department, and any regional or statewide emergency operations entities. It is important to understand how the local, regional, and statewide emergency operations command systems function. For example, during the civil unrest that followed the death of Freddie Gray from injuries sustained while in the custody of Baltimore police, the Baltimore City Health Commissioner, Dr. Leana S. Wen, was called into the Baltimore Emergency Operations Center as head of one of the lead agencies involved in response to destruction of health clinics and pharmacies. Dr. Wen was able to initiate alternative means for vulnerable residents to receive their medications and other health services with hospitals in the community until a direct prescription and clinic support services were reestablished through the health department. Supporting patients with chronic conditions helped prevent many patients from health care crises that could have led to emergency room visits and inpatient stays.

Case in Point
Extreme Weather Event: Hospitals in Baltimore and Clarksburg, West Virginia, Cope with Heavy Snowfall Blanketing the Area

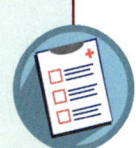

Preparation

As news of the gathering storm began to reach them, leaders at Highland Clarksburg Hospital, a 150 bed psychiatric hospital in north central West Virginia, began to monitor the weather forecasts. It soon became clear that they were in for a major weather event. By Monday of that week, January 18, 2016, the National Weather Service was forecasting the area would receive between 10 and 18 inches of snow. That morning hospital leaders activated their Emergency Operations Plan and began preparations to ready the hospital for the storm.

Senior leadership was alerted through a phone tree, and the emergency management team began to activate its contacts with the state police, county authorities, and the federal government. Leaders activated the radio network that connects hospitals in West Virginia. They also began participating in regular conference calls that included state police and the Department of Homeland Security. Hospital staff began to account for critical supplies, in case the hospital should become isolated and unreachable due to impassible roads. This included food and water, linens, diesel fuel for generators, and salt for ice. Arrangements were also made to pick up staff members or take them home by hospital personnel.

Meanwhile, the emergency management team at the University of Maryland Medical Center in Baltimore had also been tracking the storm for days. Drawing on their experiences during a major blizzard in 2010, the team initiated plans to cope with the snowfall and ensure adequate staffing.

Response

At ten o'clock on the morning of January 22 the Incident Command Center was opened, and it was determined that all nonessential staff at Highland Clarksburg Hospital were to be released at 1:00 P.M. Those who stayed (clinical, maintenance, and dietary) were told that they would likely be staying through the weekend, as the predicted amounts of snow were likely to prevent traffic in or out of the hospital. Arrangements were made to feed and house staff and patients during the duration of the storm. Nearly 50 staff stayed through the storm, and the dietary staff provided meals and snacks for all patients and staff.

Conference calls were set up twice a day, during which hospital officials and others were given detailed information about the storm's progress, time bands and predictions for snowfall, and other critical updates. Hospital leaders were also able to communicate their needs to local authorities. Meanwhile, staff kept the hospital's more than 65 patients occupied with exercise, crafts, and other indoor activities. The staff placed an emphasis on maintaining normal functioning and normal routines.

(continued on page 20)

The University of Maryland Medical Center had activated its incident command the previous day and opened its command center and began coordinated preparations for the coming snow. These included topping off all supplies, making arrangements to provide temporary housing within the hospital for staff, and messaging staff to make arrangements so each could work his or her assigned shifts. The planning paid off; by Friday evening downtown Baltimore and the surrounding region was snowed in and virtually no one was coming to or leaving the medical center. Having provided these services in the previous blizzard for a week or more, the organization handled the three-day emergency with relative ease.

Challenges

By Sunday morning, June 24, the storm had blown through, leaving nearly 20 inches of snow in its wake. Staff at Highland Clarksburg Hospital had been working throughout the storm to clear the snow using hospital snow removal vehicles. "Maybe the biggest problem," said Highland Clarksburg CEO Mike Casdorph, "was where to put all that snow." With no more new snow falling, snow removal began to catch up. Though one of the hospital's snow removers broke down, help was procured through a memorandum of understanding with the Veterans Administration.

Some staffing issues arose due to impassible roads preventing staff from traveling from home to work, but many either were able to make it in on their own or were brought in by hospital vehicles. Staffing levels remained adequate at all times. In fact, due to solid planning and leadership, good luck, and good work by staff, Casdorph says, "I doubt many of our patients even noticed [the emergency], other than there was a lot of snow falling outside."

Similarly, incident commanders at the University of Maryland talked with pride of the way their staff were able to ride out the storm without missing a beat, operationally speaking. They credited this not only to their experience with severe weather events, but to having a large cross-functional hospital incident command team whose members really like working together and who practice/use the incident command regularly.

Working with Other Health Care Organizations

To ensure a coordinated response to an emergency, it is important to establish contact, build relationships, and develop health care partnerships before an emergency occurs. It is essential to cultivate relationships with industry groups, state and regional associations, and organizations based on treatment specialties, such as burn treatment centers, trauma centers, or pediatric intensive care facilities, during an emergency. This alliance, or coalition, gives organizations the opportunity to plan and prepare together while combining resources. Resources to help with the formation and nurturing of such coalitions are available on the US Department of Health and Human Services' Technical Resources, Assistance Center, and Inform0ation Exchange (TRACIE) website at https://asprtracie.hhs.gov/technical-resources/21/Healthcare-Coalition-Development-and-Organization.

Coalition leaders—usually emergency managers—coordinate the participating organizations under county, state, or regional ICS. They also act as a liaison between the health care coalition's member organizations and their community emergency partners; organizations that may be competitors in conventional times develop effective teams that can communicate and respond in coordinated efforts during disasters.

One such coalition—Mutual Aid Coordinating Entity (MACE)—was developed through the efforts of 31 hospitals in the Hudson Valley region of New York. Members of MACE understood that a system of partnering with other health care organizations would provide the extended capabilities needed to face a true emergency. Coalition leaders coordinated regular emergency exercises, such as simulating a plane crash. They also offered training for situations such as hazardous materials accidents and hospital fires.* Joint exercises such as these demonstrate the potential capabilities of coalitions to effectively address complex regional disasters.

Strengthening Relationships with Suppliers

Before an emergency, organizations should assess their relationships with suppliers and make sure those companies can deliver supplies during an emergency. This includes discussing with a supplier the ways in which that company will get supplies to the health care organization and how many other health care organizations the company has agreed to supply. If a supplier has only one route or method for delivering supplies to an organization, for example, the organization and the supplier should develop a contingency plan for getting supplies to the organization should that route be compromised. Establishing an alternative route isn't the only contingency plan organizations should work out with suppliers. It is also a prudent move to contact suppliers out of the local area or even out of the state/region as a backup plan; local suppliers might experience the same issues (flooding, lack of staff, loss of power, and so on) as the organization during a localized disaster. Suppliers might be prepared and ready to deliver supplies from preloaded trucks, but that doesn't help organizations much if the drivers of those trucks are evacuated and can't transport the expected emergency provisions.

Discussions with suppliers should also include alternate supplies if a particular item is unavailable. For example, if a particular flu vaccine is unavailable, is there another alternate pharmaceutical that may be utilized? During the H1N1 outbreak, respirators, gowns, and gloves were in short supply internationally. Items with long delivery, chronic shortage, or high demand should be reviewed with team members charged with evaluating supplies.

Planning for 96 Hours

As mentioned above, Joint Commission standards require leaders to plan for how the hospital can continue to provide services safely during a disaster for at least 96 hours without local community support. This requires organizations not only to actively monitor critical supplies, but to dynamically re-allocate resources, modify services, or otherwise adjust response activities as the emergency evolves. Should an organization determine that it cannot provide care safely for at least 96 hours, alternate response strategies, including evacuation, may be implemented in a timely manner. Criteria for determining how an organization determined its ratings should be documented. During an event, the 96-hour documentation

---

* The MACE Standard Operating Guidelines, from NorMet (Northern Metropolitan Hospital Association), were written by and for hospitals that are signatories to the Mutual Aid Agreement.

may prove useful by incident command for decision making. Like many organizations, Mercy Health in Cincinnati developed a tool that organizations may use to track on an ongoing basis their resources and their ability to project their capability to provide service for at least 96 hours (*see* Figure 2-4 on page 23).

Addressing an Evacuation

One aspect of emergency management with which organizations often struggle is evacuation. Although it should be considered only as a last resort, circumstances may dictate that it is the only possible action to keep patients and staff safe. Organizations that choose to stay open during an emergency must have plans to be self-sufficient for at least 96 hours. If staying open for 96 hours is not possible, the organizations should have plans for closing or evacuating after a certain period of time. The need for community coordination and planning prior to an emergency is of paramount importance. If necessary, alternative sites for patient care must be established in advance, and confirmation of the type and number of ambulances available for transport must be closely monitored. The phasing of which patients are evacuated at what time is dependent on patient acuity, the staff available to evacuate with the patient, and so forth. Attentiveness to the timing of communitywide evacuation orders is essential due to its impact on how a hospital or nursing care center transports evacuated patients and what routes it can use to get them to alternative sites. Organizations need to plan for every eventuality, including the prospect of facing emergency circumstances alone, should community partners be unable to provide anticipated assistance.

Organizations should also consider what to do when the emergency is over. They should define who has the authority to declare an emergency over and should have a specific plan that addresses the financial, staff, and patient care aspects of recovery and potential return of patients.

Incident Command Structure

The ICS refers to the combination of facilities, equipment, personnel, procedures, and communications operating within a common organizational structure and designed to aid in the management of resources during incident response. A clear command structure is not only mandated by Joint Commission standards, it is essential to efficient operations in an emergency situation. The Joint Commission does not require any specific structure; whether an organization adopts the Hospital Incident Command System (HICS) or some other community structure, the EOP must detail explicitly the process for assigning roles to staff, the reporting structure for information and decision making, and the responsibilities of staff for the six critical areas during the response and recovery phases. Figure 2-5 on page 24 provides an overview of the five functional areas of the Incident Command Structure and a sample organizational chart to help emergency planners envision how an effective incident command structure might look in practice. (*See* Figure 2-6 beginning on page 26 for an in-depth look at the responsibilities of the incident commander.)

Community Integration

As important as clarity of roles is within the organization, it is equally important that health care organizations be integrated into the broader community disaster response network. ICSs govern decision making and communication within organizations. The analogous

Figure 2-4. 96-Hour Operational Impact Chart

96-Hour Operational Impact Chart	Date		
Hours of Emergency Operations	0 1 2 4 6 8 10 12 14 16 18 20 22 24 26 28 30 32 34 36 38 40 42 44 46 48 50 52 54 56 60 64 68 72 76 80 84 88 92 96		
Normal Electrical Power Failure			
Emergency Electrical Power Failure/No Normal			
Emergency Electrical Power Failure/With Normal			
Loss Steam Boiler (Winter/Summer)			
Loss of Hot Water Boiler (Winter/Summer)			
Loss of Natural Gas			
Loss of Fuel Oil			
Loss of Both Natural Gas and Fuel Oil			
Loss of Propane			
City Water Pressure Low			
Loss of City Water Supply	Implement facility emergency water plan		
Loss of the Use of Sewer System	Implement emergency sanitation plan		
Loss of Chiller System—Cooling Season	Emergency comfort actions needed for patients / staff / visitors, fan distribution		
Loss of Chiller System—Non-Cooling Season	No adverse operations in heating months if less than 55° F		
Loss of Ability to Refill Main O2 Tank (Full)	Calculation of current supply needed as soon as possible		
Loss of Major Air Handling Equipment	Emergency comfort actions needed for patient / staff / visitors. Patient relocation possible.		
Loss of Telephone Switch	Need to implement emergency measures		
Loss of Phone Service			
Loss of Computer Server	There is a 8 hour time frame needed to implement emergency plan		
Loss of Elevator(s)			
Loss of Laundry Services			
Food and Nutrition Products			
Medication			
Sump Pump Failure			
Loss of Bulk Oxygen			
Loss Of Medical Air			
Loss of Medical Vacuum			
Loss of Nitrogen			
Loss of Trash Pickup			
Loss of Essential Transport Activities			
Loss of Morgue Space			
Loss of Paper Products			
Loss of Medical Waste Pickup			
Loss of Essential Staff			
Loss of Medical Supplies			
Hourly Facility Updates to Administration and Clinical Management	Provided by Senior Facilities Department member		
Command Center Maintains Communication with Local, County, State, & Federal Agencies	Information received distributed as appropriate		
Hourly Communications Status Provided to Administration and Clinical Management	Provided by Senior Communications Department member		
Administration and Clinical Management Evaluate Possible Patient Transfer or Discharge on an Hourly Basis	Chief Executive Officer and Chief Nursing Officer		
Hourly Resources and Assets Updates to Administration and Clinical Management	Provided by Senior Material Management Department member		
Hourly Food Services Updates to Administration	Provided by Senior Food Service Department member		
Hourly Safety and Security Updates Given to Administration and Clinical Management	Provided by Senior Security Department member		
Administration and Clinical Management Provide Information and Expectation to Staff as Needed	Chief Nursing Officer and Chief Operating Officer		
Hourly Administration and Clinical Management Assess Patient/Staff Needs	Chief Executive Officer and Chief Nursing Officer		

Green = Indicates that all patient, staff, and visitor services can continue without any discernible impact or change

Yellow = Indicates that selected patient, staff, and visitor services may be revised or terminated
It is likely that elective surgeries may be affected and some or all outpatient services may be temporarily terminated
Some conservation may be required by affected staff and patients. Visitors and visitors' hour may be limited.

Red = All incoming patients and visitors will be denied admission to the hospital. All activity will be centered around maintaining the quality of life for our patients as we proceed with the evacuation of the hospital.

Examples:
Loss of Chiller System—Non Cooling Season	No adverse operations in heating months if less than 55° F
Loss of Ability to Refill Main O2 Tank (Full)	Calculation of current supply needed as soon as possible

Evacuation/Closure of Hospital Variables
*Conservation of resources
* Possible curtailment of services
* Supplementing of resources from outside the local community
* Staged evacuation

Developed by MHP EOC PSC 8/08

Figure 2-4 helps organizations assess their ability to provide services without community support for at least 96 hours.
Source: Rita Snyder RN, MSN, NE-BC, CHSP, Mercy Health Vice President of Accreditation. Used with permission.

external structure is the National Incident Management System (NIMS). NIMS was created by the US government to help lend clarity to roles and eliminate duplicate effort and jurisdictional conflict. Hospitals and other health care organizations must establish and maintain relationships with community disaster response partners in compliance with NIMS. The Capacity Builder on page 25 describes NIMS and HICS in greater detail, and how they fit together.

Figure 2-5. **Incident Command Structure Leadership Responsibilities**

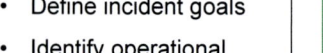

Operations	Planning	Logistics	Finance/Admin
• Establish strategy to meet incident goals • Identify specific tactics to meet operational objectives • Coordinate and execute chosen strategy and tactics	• Support command and operations in use of personnel, supplies, and equipment • Perform technical activities to maintain operational facilities and processes	• Coordinate support activities for incident planning • Coordinate support activities for contingency, long-range, and demobilization planning • Support command and operations in processing incident information • Coordinate information activities across the response system	• Support command and operations with administrative issues • Track and process incident expenses • Coordinate licensure requirements, regulatory compliance, and financial accounting issues

Figure 2-5 provides a representation of the Incident Command Structure.

Capacity Builder

The National Incident Management System[1] and the Hospital Incident Command System[2]: Two Models Help Navigate the Emergency Management Process

What Is the National Incident Management System?
- Comprehensive, nationwide, systematic all-hazards approach to incident management
- Core set of doctrine, concepts, principles, terminology, and organizational processes for all hazards
- Essential principles for a common operating picture and interoperability of communications and information management
- Standardized resource management procedures for coordination among different jurisdictions and organizations
- Scalable and applicable for all incidents

Key Benefits
- Enhances organizational and technological interoperability and cooperation
- Provides a scalable and flexible framework with universal applicability
- Enables a wide variety of organizations to participate effectively in emergency management / incident response
- Institutionalizes professional emergency management/incident response practices

What Is the Hospital Incident Command System?
- Flexible and scalable incident management system addressing planning and response needs of any size hospital with universal applicability
- Predictable chain of command with a suggested span of control
- Accountable position and team functions, including prioritized action checklists
- Common language for promoting interagency communication
- Modular design and adaptability allowing planning and management of nonemergent incidents or events
- Guidance requirements from the NIMS and accreditation agencies regarding hospital use of Incident Command System principles with community partners
- Management by objectives in which the problem encountered is evaluated, a plan to remedy the problem is identified and implemented, and resources assigned

The Hospital Incident Command System, the National Incident Management System, and Joint Commission Standards

Both HICS and NIMS can help organizations comply with The Joint Commission's Emergency Management standards. Although HICS and NIMS can be used to comply with many of the Joint Commission requirements, compliance with HICS or NIMS does not automatically mean compliance with Joint Commission requirements found in the Emergency Operations Plan standard. The Joint Commission standards offer a framework for effective emergency management, and each organization must tailor an effective program for emergency management within that framework.

REFERENCES

1. Federal Emergency Management Agency (FEMA). National Incident Management System. (Updated: May 11, 2016.) Accessed Jun 21, 2016. http://www.fema.gov/national-incident-management-system.
2. California Emergency Medical Services Authority (EMSA). *Hospital Incident Command Services Guidebook*, 5th ed. Rancho Cordova, CA: EMSA, 2014. Accessed Jun 21, 2016. http://emsa.ca.gov/media/default/HICS/HICS_Guidebook_2014_11.pdf.

Figure 2-6. Incident Commander

INCIDENT COMMANDER

Mission: Organize and direct the Hospital Command Center (HCC). Give overall strategic direction for hospital incident management and support activities, including emergency response and recovery. Approve the Incident Action Plan (IAP) for each operational period.

Position Reports to: **Executive Administration**   Command Location: _____

Position Contact Information: Phone: (____) - _____   Radio Channel: _____

Hospital Command Center (HCC): Phone: (____) - _____   Fax: (____) - _____

Position Assigned to:	Date: / /	Start: ___:___ hrs.
Signature:	Initials:	End: ___:___ hrs.
Position Assigned to:	Date: / /	Start: ___:___ hrs.
Signature:	Initials:	End: ___:___ hrs.
Position Assigned to:	Date: / /	Start: ___:___ hrs.
Signature:	Initials:	End: ___:___ hrs.

Immediate Response (0 – 2 hours)	Time	Initial
Receive appointment • Gather intelligence, information and likely impact from the sources providing event notification • Assume the role of Incident Commander and activate the Hospital Incident Command System (HICS) • Review this Job Action Sheet • Put on position identification (e.g., position vest) • Notify your usual supervisor and the Hospital Chief Executive Officer (CEO) of the incident, activation of the Hospital Command Center (HCC), and your assignment		

Assess the operational situation
• Activate the Hospital Emergency Operations Plan (EOP) and applicable Incident Specific Plans or Annexes
• Brief Command Staff on objectives and issues, including:
  o Size and complexity of the incident
  o Expectations
  o Involvement of outside agencies, stakeholders, and organizations
  o The situation, incident activities, and any special concerns
• Seek feedback and further information		

Determine the incident objectives, tactics, and assignments
• Determine incident objectives for the operational period
• Determine which Command Staff need to be activated:
  o Safety Officer
  o Liaison Officer
  o Public Information Officer
• Determine the impact on affected departments and gather additional information from the Liaison Officer
• Appoint a Planning Section Chief to develop an Incident Action Plan (IAP)
• Appoint an Operations Section Chief to provide support and direction to affected areas
• Appoint a Logistics Section Chief to provide support and direction to affected areas		

HICS 2014 | Page 1 of 5

CHAPTER 2 | The Emergency Operations Plan

Figure 2-6. **Incident Commander** (continued)

INCIDENT COMMANDER		
<ul><li>Appoint a Finance Section Chief to provide support and direction to affected areas</li><li>Determine the need for, and appropriately appoint or ensure appointment of Medical-Technical Specialists</li><li>Make assignments and distribute corresponding Job Action Sheets and position identification</li><li>Ensure hospital and key staff are notified of the activation of the Hospital Command Center (HCC)</li><li>Identify the operational period and any planned Hospital Incident Management Team (HIMT) staff shift changes</li><li>Conduct a meeting with HIMT staff to receive status reports from Section Chiefs and Command Staff to determine appropriate response and recovery levels, then set the time for the next briefing</li></ul>		
Activities<ul><li>Ensure all activated positions are documented in the Incident Action Plan (IAP) and on status boards</li><li>Obtain current patient census and status from the Planning Section Chief</li><li>Determine the need to activate surge plans based on current patient status and injury projections</li><li>If additional beds are needed, authorize a patient prioritization assessment for the purposes of designating appropriate early discharge</li><li>If applicable, receive an initial hospital damage survey report from the Operations Section Infrastructure Branch and evaluate the need for evacuation</li></ul>		
Documentation<ul><li>Incident Action Plan (IAP) Quick Start</li><li>HICS 200: Consider whether to use the Incident Action plan (IAP) Cover Sheet</li><li>HICS 201: Initiate the Incident Briefing form</li><li>HICS 204: Assign or complete the Assignment List as appropriate</li><li>HICS 207: Assign or complete the Hospital Incident Management Team (HIMT) Chart for assigned positions</li><li>HICS 213: Document all communications on a General Message Form</li><li>HICS 214: Document all key activities, actions, and decisions in an Activity Log on a continual basis</li><li>HICS 252: Distribute the Section Personnel Time Sheet to Command and Medical-Technical Specialist Staff and ensure time is recorded appropriately</li></ul>		
Resources<ul><li>Assign one or more clerical personnel from current staffing or make a request for staff to the Logistics Section Chief, if activated, to function as Hospital Command Center (HCC) recorders</li></ul>		
Communication *Hospital to complete: Insert communications technology, instructions for use and protocols for interface with external partners*		
Safety and security<ul><li>Ensure that appropriate safety measures and risk reduction activities are initiated</li><li>Ensure that HICS 215A – Incident Action Plan Safety Analysis is completed and distributed</li><li>Ensure that a hospital damage survey is completed if the incident warrants</li></ul>		

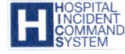

HICS 2014 | Page 2 of 5

(continued on page 28)

27

Figure 2-6. Incident Commander (continued)

INCIDENT COMMANDER

Intermediate Response (2 – 12 hours)	Time	Initial

Activities
• Transfer the Incident Commander role, if appropriate
   ○ Conduct a transition meeting to brief your replacement on the current situation, response actions, available resources and the role of external agencies in support of the hospital
   ○ Address any health, medical, or safety concerns
   ○ Address political sensitivities, when appropriate
   ○ Instruct your replacement to complete the appropriate documentation and ensure that appropriate personnel are briefed on response issues and objectives (see HICS Forms 203, 204, 214, and 215A)
• Schedule regular briefings with Hospital Incident Management Team (HIMT) staff to identify and plan to:
   ○ Ensure a patient tracking system is established and linked with appropriate outside agencies and the local Emergency Operations Center (EOC)
   ○ Develop, review, and revise the Incident Action Plan (IAP), or its elements, as needed
   ○ Approve the IAP revisions if developed by the Planning Section Chief, then ensure that the approved plan is communicated to HIMT staff
   ○ Ensure that safety measures and risk reduction activities are ongoing and re-evaluate if necessary
• Consider deploying a Public Information Officer to the local Joint Information Center (JIC), if applicable		

Documentation • HICS 214: Document all key activities, actions, and decisions in an Activity Log on a continual basis		
Resources • Authorize resources as needed or requested by Command Staff or Section Chiefs		
Communication *Hospital to complete: Insert communications technology, instructions for use and protocols for interface with external partners*		
Safety and security • Ensure that patient and personnel safety measures and risk reduction actions are followed		

Extended Response (greater than 12 hours)	Time	Initial

Activities
• Transfer the Incident Commander role, if appropriate
   ○ Conduct a transition meeting to brief your replacement on the current situation, response actions, available resources and the role of external agencies in support of the hospital
   ○ Address any health, medical, or safety concerns
   ○ Address political sensitivities, when appropriate
   ○ Instruct your replacement to complete the appropriate documentation and ensure that appropriate personnel are briefed on response issues and objectives (see HICS Forms 203, 204, 214, and 215A)
• Evaluate or re-evaluate the need for deploying a Public Information Officer to the local Joint Information Center (JIC) and a Liaison Officer to the local Emergency Operations Center (EOC), if applicable
• Ensure that an Incident Action Plan (IAP) is developed for each operational period, approved, and provided to Section Chiefs for operational period briefings
• With Section Chiefs, determine the recovery and reimbursement costs and ensure documentation of financial impact		

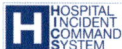

HICS 2014 | Page 3 of 5

Figure 2-6. **Incident Commander** *(continued)*

INCIDENT COMMANDER		
• Ensure staff, patient, and media briefings are being conducted regularly		
Documentation • HICS 214: Document all key activities, actions, and decisions in an Activity Log on a continual basis		
Resources • Authorize resources as needed or requested by Command Staff and Section Chiefs		
Communication *Hospital to complete: Insert communications technology, instructions for use and protocols for interface with external partners*		
Safety and security • Observe all staff and volunteers for signs of stress and inappropriate behavior and report concerns to the Safety Officer and the Logistics Section Employee Health and Well-Being Unit Leader • Provide for personnel rest periods and relief • Ensure your physical readiness through proper nutrition, water intake, rest, and stress management techniques		

Demobilization/System Recovery	Time	Initial

Activities
• Transfer the Incident Commander role, if appropriate
    o Conduct a transition meeting to brief your replacement on the current situation, response actions, available resources and the role of external agencies in support of the hospital
    o Address any health, medical, or safety concerns
    o Address political sensitivities, when appropriate
    o Instruct your replacement to complete the appropriate documentation and ensure that appropriate personnel are briefed on response issues and objectives (see HICS Forms 203, 204, 214, and 215A)
• Assess the plan developed by the Planning Section Demobilization Unit and approved by the Planning Section Chief for the gradual demobilization of the Hospital Command Center (HCC) and emergency operations according to the progression of the incident and hospital status
• Demobilize positions in the HCC and return personnel to their normal jobs as appropriate, in coordination with the Planning Section Demobilization Unit
• Brief staff, administration, and Board of Directors
• Approve notification of demobilization to the hospital staff when the incident is no longer active or can be managed using normal operations
• Participate in community and governmental meetings and other post-incident discussion and after action activities
• Ensure post-incident media briefings and hospital status updates are scheduled and conducted
• Ensure implementation of stress management activities and services for staff
• Ensure that staff debriefings are scheduled to identify accomplishments, response, and improvement issues		

Documentation • HICS 221- Demobilization Check-Out • Ensure all Hospital Command Center (HCC) documentation is provided to the Planning Section Documentation Unit		

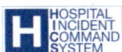

HICS 2014 | Page 4 of 5

(continued on page 30)

Figure 2-6. **Incident Commander** (continued)

INCIDENT COMMANDER

Documents and Tools

- Incident Action Plan (IAP) Quick Start
- HICS 200 - Incident Action Plan (IAP) Cover Sheet
- HICS 201 - Incident Briefing form
- HICS 203 - Organization Assignment List
- HICS 204 - Assignment List(s)
- HICS 205A - Communications List
- HICS 207: Hospital Incident Management Team (HIMT) Chart
- HICS 213 - General Message Form
- HICS 214 - Activity Log
- HICS 215A - Incident Action Plan (IAP) Safety Analysis
- HICS 221 - Demobilization Check-Out
- HICS 252 - Section Personnel Time Sheet
- HICS 258 - Hospital Resource Directory
- Hospital Emergency Operations Plan (EOP)
- Incident Specific Plans or Annexes
- Hospital organization chart
- Hospital telephone directory
- Telephone/cell phone/satellite phone/internet/amateur radio/2-way radio for communication

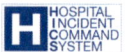

HICS 2014 | Page 5 of 5

Figure 2-6 identifies incident command management and support activities.

Source: California Emergency Medical Services Authority. Incident Commander. 2014. Accessed Jun 21, 2016. http://emsa.ca.gov/media/default/HICS/JAS/Release%201/Command/Incident%20Commander_2.pdf.

IN SUMMARY

- The first step in preparedness is identifying and evaluating risk. A thorough and thoughtful hazard vulnerability analysis is essential.

- Create an EOP to outline response to the most likely and greatest threats.

- Cultivate relationships with other health care providers, public health, first responders (fire, police, EMS), vendors, suppliers, public utilities, relevant government agencies, and other community partners. Coordinate disaster response planning with outside partners.

- Use an incident command structure to create clear lines of authority for situational awareness, efficient communication, effective decision making, and coordinated response.

REFERENCE

1. US Department of Health and Human Services. Office of the Assistant Secretary for Preparedness and Response (ASPR). *Healthcare Preparedness Capabilities: National Guidance for Healthcare System Preparedness.* Washington, DC: ASPR, 2012. Accessed Jun 21, 2016. http://www.phe.gov/Preparedness/planning/hpp/reports/Documents/capabilities.pdf.

Special Report
"Worst-Case Scenario": Planning for Crisis Standards of Care

In 2012 the federal government required the 62 jurisdictions that receive federal emergency management funding to develop crisis standards of care (CSC) in collaboration with the hospitals and other medical and mental health providers in their states, municipalities, and territories. CSC are designed to establish an integrated systems-level response to a mass-casualty event.[1] Leading up to this mandate, the US Department of Health and Human Services (HHS) had turned to the Institute of Medicine to research and develop guidance to support decision making on the allocation of scarce medical resources.[1]

The *crisis standards of care* represent a substantial change in usual health care operations and the level of care it is possible to deliver, which is made necessary by a pervasive (for example, pandemic influenza) or catastrophic (for example, earthquake, hurricane) disaster. This change in the level of care delivered is justified by specific circumstances and is formally declared by a state government, which recognizes that crisis operations will be in effect for a sustained period. The formal declaration that crisis standards of care are in operation enables specific legal/regulatory powers and protections for health care providers in the necessary tasks of allocating and using scarce medical resources and implementing alternate care facility operations.[2]

This information served as the basis for the HHS policy, which requires each state to implement the CSC framework.[2] "The goal of the CSC is to help organizations and communities plan for how to move along the continuum from providing conventional care, to a contingency response, to a crisis response," says Lynne Bergero, MHSA, project director for the Department of Standards and Survey Methodology at The Joint Commission. "While all accredited organizations have a plan in place to respond to various contingencies—as per the Joint Commission Emergency Management standards—the crisis standards of care prompt organizations to look beyond those plans and anticipate the absolute worst-case scenario; in other words, when the organization is overwhelmed by a mass-casualty event affecting the entire community."

Five Key Principles of CSC
Health care organizations around the country are still at varying stages of developing CSC. By starting to think about this framework now, organizations can begin to sift through all the considerations that go along with responding to a catastrophic situation. Five key principles underlie CSC[1]:

1. A strong ethical grounding that enables a process deemed equitable and just based on its transparency, consistency, proportionality, and accountability
2. Integrated and ongoing community and provider engagement, education, and communication
3. The necessary legal authority and legal environment in which CSC can be ethically and optimally implemented
4. Clear indicators, triggers, and lines of responsibility
5. Evidence-based clinical processes and operations

Planning for contingencies that involve large numbers of seriously ill or injured patients, with limited access to resources or facilities is a daunting task. However, organizations can adapt strategies that can help navigate the complexities and help them formulate a plan. The Institute of Medicine offers a full suite of documents that describe CSC planning in depth. This Special Report is intended to help hospitals and other health care facilities with the complex process of initiating the dialog about crisis standards of care within their organizations.

A Strong Ethical Grounding

At its simplest formulation, during a mass-casualty event affecting an entire region, a health care organization may have 60 patients to treat but only enough space, supplies, and staff to effectively treat 40. What kind of treatment do you give? To which patients? For how long? Planning for CSC by definition involves sensitive and difficult decisions concerning the allocation of scarce medical resources. Staff values regarding providing the best care possible for their patients will be at the top of their concerns. Planning for CSC requires leaders, emergency managers, clinicians, and operations and support staff to work through these ethical and allocation issues in advance, ideally with the ongoing participation of an ethicist, in a framework of principles that includes transparency, consistency, and fairness. Organizations beginning this internal discussion within their health care coalitions and with members of the patient populations they serve should refer to the extensive body of medical ethics literature, and work with a health care ethicist to support exploration of the potential ethical concerns of staff at all levels.

Provider and Community Engagement and Education

Organization leaders should provide orientation to their staff on CSC and their purpose. Not every staff member will be involved in implementing CSC during a disaster, but staff should be included in CSC planning discussions. Emergency physicians and hospitalists, pediatric advanced practice nurses and hospice nurses, pharmacists, psychiatrists, respiratory therapists—and provider types across the health care continuum—are on the front lines of care and clinical decision making; their representation on internal planning efforts will provide essential perspective to the organization's CSC planning.

Likewise, organizations should already be working with their community to plan for contingencies. CSC planning guides hospitals and health care organizations to plan together around key issues, such as the following:
- Designation of specific facilities for specific response needs
- Proactive identification and care coordination for vulnerable populations
- Crisis risk communication strategies regarding the allocation of scarce resources

Organizations that participate in their community-based or regional exercises benefit from opportunities to test and refine their response plans with coalition partners and stakeholders.

(continued on page 34)

Legal Authority and Framework

Local, state, and federal standards and regulations, as well as some Joint Commission Emergency Management (EM) and Leadership (LD) standards, support organizations in working with their staff, government authorities, and other stakeholders to proactively plan for response to and recovery from catastrophic events. In addition, several national organizations such as the American College of Emergency Physicians, the US Department of Veterans Affairs, the Emergency Nurses Association, the American College of Healthcare Executives, and the American College of Chest Physicians have published recommendations to support clinical processes and decision making related to the allocation of scarce medical resources.

In planning for CSC, health care organization leaders should be aware of the legal and regulatory frameworks that encompass issues related to disasters and potential CSC situations. Different states are at various points along the road to CSC development. For example, California, Colorado, Massachusetts, and New York—as well as several other states—have made progress in developing procedures and protocols that reflect the CSC's intent. Additional states are just starting to lay the groundwork, convening committees that include emergency response organizations, hospitals and other health care facilities, state agencies, and additional stakeholders.

Organizations also have to work through the legal issues surrounding crisis care, asking questions of their legal advisors and state authorities related to concerns such as the following:
- Alternate use of facilities and any related licensure issues
- Mutual aid agreements to expand surge capacity
- Scope of clinical practice and credentialing
- Legal liability for health care workers
- Federal waivers related to applicable laws, such as the Emergency Medical Treatment and Active Labor Act, the Health Insurance Portability and Accountability Act, and other regulations

Development of Indicators and Triggers

Leaders and staff need to discuss within their organizations and health care coalitions the indicators and triggers for shifting from conventional care to contingency care to crisis care. Joint Commission standards require organization leaders to maintain situational awareness and adjust response actions as an emergency evolves and the organization shifts from conventional care to contingency operations. CSC planning requires that organizations go further to expand on their existing indicators and triggers to address transitions from contingency to crisis situations. These indicators may at a minimum be a declared disaster by the governor, along with catastrophic utility system failures, structural damage, communication system failures, inadequate use of space for safe triage or surgeries, and critical shortage of essential equipment or supplies. In planning for CSC, the health care organization reviews and discusses with its coalition and broader community stakeholders what the likely triggers might be.

Evidence-Based Clinical Processes and Operations

Implementing policies and protocols to move toward the CSC framework is a complex and long-term endeavor, requiring attention not only to operations, facilities, and clinical issues but also to legal and cultural changes related to how care is delivered.

The Joint Commission's EM standards cover the range of contingency planning and can serve as a good foundation for organization leaders to use to move the organization through key areas of the CSC framework. For example, organization leaders may convene the stakeholders, managers, or teams currently involved in EM planning and determine together how to prioritize CSC planning activities in a phased approach over a 24-month period.

A clinical review process or committee can consider planning issues, staff education, and staff support related to the full spectrum of clinical questions. Examples of key issues include the following[3]:
- Awareness of surveillance, reporting, testing, and quarantine mandates
- Awareness of the organization's shift to CSC based on triggers
- Changes to triage and treatment processes
- Providing palliative care
- Communication and support needs of patients and families
- Communication and support needs of physicians, nurses, and clinical and non-clinical staff and leaders

Health care organizations should periodically carry out risk assessments as well as evaluate their policies and procedures to find opportunities for improvement. Opportunities for practice, such as drills and simulations, can help identify deficiencies as well as reinforce rarely implemented policies for staff. Another key area of Joint Commission EM standards that will help organizations incorporate the CSC framework relates to exercises. Most health care organizations will conduct at least two emergency management drills per year, with at least one involving a surge of patients and an escalating scenario in which the community cannot support the organization.

REFERENCES

1. Institute of Medicine. *Crisis Standards of Care: A Toolkit for Indicators and Triggers*. Washington, DC: National Academies Press, 2013. Accessed Jun 21, 2016. http://download.nap.edu/cart/download.cgi?record_id=18338.
2. US Department of Health and Human Services, Public Health Emergency. Crisis Standards of Care: A Systems Framework for Catastrophic Disaster Response. Hick J, Stroud C. Dec 18, 2012. Accessed Jun 21, 2016. http://www.phe.gov/coi/Documents/IOM%20CSC%20Briefing%20to%20OPEO%20Dec%2018%202012.pdf.
3. Institute of Medicine. *Crisis Standards of Care: A Systems Framework for Catastrophic Disaster Response*. Washington, DC: National Academies Press, 2012. Accessed Jun 21, 2016. http://download.nap.edu/cart/download.cgi?record_id=13351.

CHAPTER 3

Establishing and Facilitating Communications

STANDARDS FOCUS

EM.02.01.01 The organization has an Emergency Operations Plan.

EM.02.02.01 As part of its Emergency Operations Plan, the organization prepares for how it will communicate during emergencies.

AT A GLANCE
- Deciding who communicates with whom
- Planning communication and alert systems
- Using technology
- Planning for communication system failures

WHO IS INVOLVED?
- Organization leaders
- Department and/or unit managers
- Patients and their families
- Information management staff
- Public information officer
- Safety officer
- Security chief
- Outside agencies (law enforcement, emergency medical services [EMS], fire, local and regional emergency operations teams, and so on)
- Vendors and suppliers
- Other health care facilities and organizations
- Alternative care sites

Why Is This Critical?

The ability of organization leaders and staff to communicate with one another is important at any time in health care operations. It is particularly important during a crisis. Planning in advance what information will be shared and with whom, as well as what information will be shared with the public and how, is critical to effective response and helps to reduce confusion and anxiety. Health care organizations need to determine in advance how they will notify staff, outside agencies, and, when necessary, suppliers, vendors, and the media when they begin emergency operations. To maintain situational awareness during emergencies and to facilitate decision making, organization leaders need to receive and communicate accurate information as quickly and efficiently as possible. Clearly defining the channels of communication within the organization and with outside entities saves time and effort in an emergency. Organizations can and should use technology to facilitate communication and cope with primary systems failure. This facet of communication can help make sure that those who need information will receive it in a timely fashion—even when conditions worsen or unforeseen events arise.

Key Planning Concepts for Communications

Communication is fundamental to successful day-to-day operations of health care organizations and becomes even more crucial during crisis situations. In any emergency situation, organizations must quickly and clearly communicate a tremendous amount of information. Conversely, some emergency situations will be characterized by lack of information or conflicting information. Having a strategy for sorting through, analyzing, and synthesizing the available information will help managers decide what information to share and with whom.

Emergency Communication Processes

When designing an emergency communication strategy, organization leaders need to be able to answer these questions:

- Who will be communicating with whom?
- How will the communication take place?
- What is the plan if the primary communication systems fail?

Leaders should clearly outline emergency communications procedures in the Emergency Operations Plan (EOP) and emphasize coordination in communication outreach. When an actual emergency occurs, the organization activates its incident command center. The incident commander takes the lead in managing the emergency as it unfolds and addressing each of the six critical areas of emergency management. The organization must notify staff and any relevant outside authorities that it has triggered its EOP. If applicable, it will need to notify suppliers and vendors of the situation and inform them of immediate critical needs. Those vendors need to inform the organization of any problems or potential shortages. Staff and patients need to be kept up to date on evolving or escalating emergency conditions. In addition, the organization may need to distribute information to the media on facility conditions and available services. The organization may need to notify local authorities if it is going to curtail services, with details to be communicated to patients and the community as necessary through its website and traditional and social media.

Who Communicates an Emergency?

In light of these challenges, an organization's EOP must designate people in advance to handle communications with specific entities or individuals. The incident commander will assess the situation and, with the support of the public information officer (PIO), determine the best way to communicate the relevant information. The PIO or a designated spokesperson can coordinate with the crisis communications team. The goal of the crisis communications team is to pull together as much information as possible about the incident. The team will then determine what information should be released, the timing of the release, the mode of communication to be used, and the recipients of that information. Communication with external partners is critical to ensure consistent messaging. Their actions will keep the families of staff and patients and the community at large apprised of developments. (*See* "Capacity Builder" on page 39.) They will also brief the media about the incident and its scope and effects on the community. Security leadership can work with law enforcement and other authorities. Clinical leaders can work with emergency medical services (EMS) to coordinate preparations for a patient surge or delivery of medical equipment to disaster sites, if needed.

It is critically important that the first time the community PIO and health care organization's PIO meet is not during a disaster or emergent event. Organizations may consider attending or hosting an annual PIO meeting to introduce themselves and determine under what circumstances the community PIO or the organizations' PIO will take the lead in communicating details of an event. In general, the organization must inform all concerned parties, in a timely fashion, that the EOP is in effect. It will give details on where people should be and explain to them what they will need to do. Also, ongoing communication will enable a hospital to continuously track its ability to continue delivering services throughout the 96-hour window, as required by Joint Commission standards.

How Is Information Communicated?

The use of contact lists for each category of contact will help to make sure that all relevant parties are contacted and that everyone is kept in the loop. The organization must have a plan in place detailing how it will contact staff, patients and their families, relevant government

Capacity Builder

Crisis Communications

It is important that the crisis communications teams at health care organizations be proactive in their information strategy to preserve their ability to manage an emergency and maintain public confidence. For instance, officials at the University of Nebraska Medical Center's Biocontainment Unit worked closely with local media to allay public fears over the facility's ability to provide care and treatment safely to Ebola patients there. They were transparent about plans for transportation and infection control and forthcoming with clear and accurate information about the disease and the risks to employees and the public at large. The following is a list of questions for creating a crisis communications strategy that will help organizations deliver a clear and useful message to the public[1]:

1. At what point should crisis communications be initiated? Create a threshold that takes into account the threat to the organization, its employees, and the public at large, as well as threats to public confidence in the organization and the organization's ability to manage the emergency.

2. Who are the audiences and what is the required timing for the communication? Clinical and administrative leaders should identify the critical audiences, both internal and external.

3. Who is on the crisis communications team? Planning for the crisis communications strategy is the responsibility of a team that may include marketing and communications leaders, organizational leaders, the incident commander, designated spokespersons, information technology personnel, and others.

4. Who will deliver the message? It is important to designate and train spokespersons ahead of time.

5. How will the message be delivered? Depending on the audience, an organization may disseminate its message over an internal website, internal or external social media, traditional media, or another means. The crisis communications management team can consider how different crisis scenarios might best be addressed through different communications challenges.

6. Can certain scenarios be addressed with statements prepared ahead of time? Communications templates and prewritten statements can save time and effort in a crisis.

7. How can the plan be improved? As with any other aspect of emergency preparedness, drilling and assessment are key to improving the plan in advance of a crisis.

REFERENCE

1. Jarrard Inc. Creating a Hospital Crisis Communication Plan. Fox K. Apr 23, 2012. Accessed Jun 21, 2016. http://jarrardinc.com/jack-of-all-trades/2012/04/creating-a-hospital-crisis-communication-plan/.

agencies, community partners, the media, suppliers and vendors, and alternative care sites. This plan must designate how the contact should be made and by whom. The crisis communications team must determine the information to be conveyed and solicited and the backup technology and systems to be initiated in the event of a primary communication systems failure. If wireless provider systems become overloaded and are unable to meet the demands of an emergency situation, the team must provide an alternate plan for contacting staff who may be off site or away from their homes. This backup plan needs to identify individuals both within and without the organization to coordinate local emergency teams' operations.

Communication Channels

Within each of these channels of communication the organization must keep accurate contact information and have plans governing what information is released or communicated. Without the distribution of clear and credible information, health care staff, patients and their families, and the community as a whole can become increasingly stressed as speculation abounds. Increasingly, organizations are leveraging social media and Web-based applications to facilitate both internal and external communications. The use of disaster blogs and social media posts can be useful in disseminating information quickly to the public and the media, which can reduce the volume of incoming calls. Web-based applications can be used for such activities as tracking supplies and updating patient censuses in real time, allowing regional coalitions to coordinate response to patient surge.

Leaders, Staff, and Licensed Independent Practitioners

The EOP will contain a plan for notifying leadership, department heads, clinical and nursing staff, licensed independent practitioners, and information management staff. Staff are briefed through the incident command structure as they shift from their normal operational roles to their emergency response modes. The crisis communications team will implement systems for communicating information and instructions as the situation evolves.

The EOP will have in place a contact list for all emergency response staff, organization, and clinical leadership, and other critical positions at the organization's incident command center. The contact list could include addresses, home and cell phone numbers, e-mail addresses, and contact information for next of kin. Organizational and emergency response leaders may also keep copies of the contact lists in their offices and homes. (*See* Figure 3-1 on page 41 for a sample contact list for key hospital staff.)

Community Collaboration

During an emergency, organizations may release limited information to the PIO, the media, and the general public. First and foremost, however, they must respect their patients' rights to privacy. They may reveal patients' conditions and locations only if patients provide their names and have not requested that their information remain confidential. Even then, their health conditions may only be described with single-word responses, such as the following:
- Undetermined: Patients are waiting for assessment.
- Good: Vital signs are stable and patients are conscious.
- Fair: Vital signs are stable but patients may be uncomfortable.
- Serious: Vital signs are unstable and patients are critically ill.
- Critical: Vital signs are unstable and patients may be unconscious.

The only other situations in which organizations may release patient information might be to alert law enforcement agencies of health and safety threats or to release news of patient deaths, and even then, only after they have notified next of kin.

Source: Health First. Brevard County Public Information Officers: Contact and Communication Guidelines. Rockledge, FL: Health First, 2011.

CHAPTER 3 | Establishing and Facilitating Communications

Figure 3-1. **Sample Communications List**

HICS 205A–Communications List

1. Incident Name

2. Operational Period (#   )
Date: From _____ To: _____
Time: From _____ To: _____

3. Internal Contacts

Assignment/Name	Radio Ch #/ Frequency	Phone	Fax	Email	Mobile Phone	Pager	Identification Number of Device Issued/ Comments

4. Special Instructions

(continued on page 42)

41

Figure 3-1. **Sample Communications List** *(continued)*

HICS 205A–Communications List							
5. External Contacts							
Agency/Assignment/ Name	Radio Ch #/ Frequency	Phone	Fax	Email	Mobile Phone	Pager	Identification Number of Device Issued/ Comments

6. Special Instructions

7. Prepared by Communications Unit Leader

Print Name _____ Signature _____

Date/Time _____ Facility _____

Figure 3-1 shows a sample communications list organizations might use to ensure their ability to reach relevant staff and community partners.

Source: California Emergency Medical Services Authority. HICS 205A—Communications List. 2014. Accessed Jun 21, 2016. http://www.emsa.ca.gov/Media/default/HICS/Forms/HICS%20205A-Communications%20List.docx.

Setting Spotlight

Nursing Care Centers

Before any emergency, an organization's Emergency Operations Plan (EOP) will develop critical communications processes for incident command staff to reach a wide range of groups: organization staff, local agencies, community partners, vendors and suppliers, the media, and the community at large—patient families among them.

Patients must be kept informed as well. In certain settings, such as nursing care centers, residents who are separated from family members may be particularly fearful about new and confusing situations. They will require practical information, such as where to go in the facility and what to expect regarding their physical needs. They also will need to understand their roles and responsibilities. Perhaps most importantly, they will need reassurance.

One of the ways organizations can meet these needs is through supplying pastoral counseling to residents. Individuals handle fear and anxiety differently, and a crisis may compound those emotions. Providing spiritual resources will meet the needs of many residents. While staff initiate emergency response protocols, residents may find it upsetting or difficult to make sense of circumstances. Spiritual advisors may offer a source of calm to residents in the midst of an unsettling situation.

These individuals may be part of the organization or belong to an outside group coordinated in the EOP to assist in emergency scenarios. They can offer comfort and care to residents across a broad range of cultural, societal, and religious backgrounds and needs. Whatever their own beliefs, spiritual staff need to respect differences in the beliefs of residents and be prepared to offer hope and a sense of calm to all who need it. They will need to know how to listen without judging what they hear. They will offer an opportunity for residents to voice their concerns and hear the concerns of others.

If advisors find themselves unable to respond appropriately to some of the residents' worries, they may need to seek assistance from regular staff. Taking residents' concerns seriously and offering them a safe harbor in which to be heard will go a long way toward reassuring them and encouraging an orderly response to an emergency situation.

Source: National Voluntary Organizations Active in Disaster (National VOAD). National VOAD Disaster Spiritual Care Guidelines. Alexandria, VA: National VOAD, 2014. Accessed Jun 21, 2016. http://www.nvoad.org/mdocs-posts/national-voad-disaster-spiritual-care-guidelines/.

After contact is made with leadership across all departments, notification to the rest of the staff can be communicated via coded alarm systems, text messages, e-mails, or through posts to staff-only intranet or social media groups. Additional communication or updates can use similar methods, or other methods such as public address announcements, posted placards, color-coded emergency signs or lights, and dry-erase boards. Communication methods should communicate critical information to staff as the situation evolves—without upsetting patients unduly. Also, face-to-face communication, in the form of periodic meetings and of department heads or their designees making rounds and briefing staff, is a good way to disseminate accurate and timely information and to reduce confusion. Face-to-face communication also carries the benefit of giving staff the sense that leadership is available to convey information both down and up the chain of command.

External Authorities

Many emergencies require the organization to establish and maintain communication with external authorities, including local emergency management authorities, EMS, the Federal Emergency Management Agency (FEMA), the Centers for Disease Control and Prevention (CDC), law enforcement, and others. The community's incident command structure will direct communication with external state and federal authorities (such as the National Guard and FEMA) to maximize efficiency of response and minimize duplication and jurisdictional conflicts. The organization's incident command center maintains a list of agencies and individuals that should be contacted during the course of an emergency. The incident command staff will establish and maintain contact with external agencies. Through this process, the organization will notify its response partners that it has initiated the EOP and will exchange current and relevant information as the situation progresses.

Patients and Families

It is important to provide patients and family members with information about the emergency as quickly as practicable. First and foremost, they need to know that an emergency is occurring, and they need to be instructed and/or guided by staff regarding measures under way for their safety.

Following the initial notification, staff can provide patients and families with updates as needed as the response progresses, particularly if the emergency damages the facility or requires changes in patient care, treatment, or service. Communicating effectively with patients and their families can reduce anxiety. Staff can keep patients calm and inform them

Capacity Builder

The purpose of an initial press statement is to answer the basic questions who, what, where, when. This statement should provide any guidance possible at the given point in time, express the organization's concern about the situation, and explain how additional information will be communicated. When possible, the statement should give phone numbers or contacts for more information or assistance. *What follows is a template meant only to provide guidance. This template will not work for every situation.*

FOR IMMEDIATE RELEASE
CONTACT: (name of contact)
PHONE: (number of contact)
Date of release: (date)
Headline—Insert your primary message to the public
Dateline (your location)—
Two or three sentences describing current situation. Insert quote from an official spokesperson demonstrating leadership and concern for any victims. Insert actions currently being taken.
List actions that *will be* taken.
List information on possible reactions of the public and ways citizens can help. Insert quote from an official spokesperson providing reassurance.
List contact information, ways to get more information, and other resources.

Source: Centers for Disease Control and Prevention. CERC Template for News Release. Accessed Jun 21, 2016. http://emergency.cdc.gov/cerc/resources/pdf/cercnewsrelease.pdf.

Vulnerable Populations

Managing Communications with Patients of Limited English Proficiency

Communication in an emergency is always challenging, and the more so when a facility is faced with an influx of patients with limited English proficiency (LEP). To treat patients effectively, staff need to understand what patients are trying to tell them, and staff need to be able to communicate information to patients about their condition and treatment options. In addition, parents or assigned parties of minor or incapacitated patients may also communicate in a language other than English, and they will need to understand information about treatment to make decisions.

Joint Commission standards require that patient care and treatment information be communicated to patients in a manner and language they can understand. Many organizations contract interpreter services to fill this need and use written materials translated into the languages used by their patient populations. Another way of addressing this issue is to maintain a diverse and multilingual staff, providing some staff members with training to work as interpreters with LEP patients and families. Human resources professionals can factor language capabilities into hiring decisions, in an attempt to match the organization's capabilities to the linguistic diversity in its community. Some of those hired may become licensed interpreters as part of their professional development.

Ultimately, however, during a large influx of patients, the combined internal and contracted interpreting capacity of any organization may be overwhelmed. In such situations, emergency managers may want to reach out to health care coalitions to identify additional interpreter services. In addition, several agencies have developed resources that support communication in multiple languages during disasters:

ECHO Minnesota develops multi-language resources to foster health and well-being among the diverse communities living in Minnesota. In cooperation with the Minnesota Department of Health, ECHO has developed a tool entitled "Communicating Without English in an Emergency Planning Template" that can be adapted for use in other states. The tool is available at http://www.echominnesota.org/sites/default/files/Planning%20Template%20-%20Fillable%20FINAL.pdf.

The US Department of Homeland Security has developed several resources to support communication in disasters with LEP populations. The "I Speak" posters help with initiating discussion with new patients and determining what type of interpreter may be needed. They can be accessed at https://www.dhs.gov/xlibrary/assets/crcl/crcl-i-speak-booklet.pdf.

The National Resource Center on Advancing Emergency Preparedness for Culturally Diverse Communities hosts a website that contains a range of resources that support disaster preparedness and communication with diverse populations at http://www.diversitypreparedness.org/.

Translation and interpreter services are only one element of preparedness for LEP patient populations. How various LEP communities receive notifications of emergencies and ongoing updates may vary. Hospitals and health care coalitions may consider alternative media sources, such as language-specific radio stations and community newspapers, for ongoing communication regarding response and recovery efforts, or partnering with schools, faith-based organizations, and small-business networks to help disseminate disaster-related information.

Community Collaboration

Addressing the Media
When speaking with the media, consider the following tips:
- Answer questions directly, without giving more information than necessary.
- Look for opportunities in the interview to share key approved messages.
- Remain calm. If a reporter gets aggressive, stay focused on the question at hand and try to answer to the best of your ability.
- Never say, "No comment." It is OK to say, "I don't know."
- Never flatly refuse to give information. Explain why the information is not available (for example, patient confidentiality).
- Remember that anything you say during the course of the conversation could appear in print, over the airwaves, or online. There is no such thing as "off the record."
- If a reporter uses negative language, do not repeat it and do not repeat the question.
- Avoid arguing with a news reporter about a story.
- Do not let a reporter put words in your mouth. Clarify comments when necessary.
- Repeating key messages is acceptable. Sometimes a reporter needs to hear a message several times and in several ways to capture the full message.

of any developments. They can also inform family members if patient care is affected or if patients are relocated to other health care facilities or alternative care sites.

In addition, the organization can use its communication systems to disseminate critical information. For instance, in the event of an infectious disease outbreak, bioterrorist attack, or radiological event, the organization can help spread accurate information about risks, measures to prevent exposure, and first aid and treatment information, as well as information about where to go or where to take patients in the event of exposure.

It may be useful to set up one or more hotlines to be made available to patient and staff family members. Through prerecorded messages, family members can access information critical to their particular situations. As circumstances change, the organization can update information as necessary. Information on individual patients and their conditions will be provided only on a case-by-case basis by the patient's nurse or physician and then only if the request for information comes from an immediate family member with a right to know the information requested. The planning team should decide, in advance, whenever possible, what information will be released to family members consistent with HIPAA.

Organizations might also choose to have available an on-site family information center in which pastoral care workers, social workers, case managers, and other personnel can provide information and support for family and friends waiting for information on the condition of disaster victims. They can have on hand fact sheets addressing how to handle the stress that comes as part of an emergency.

Community, Media, and Social Media
Not all emergencies require implementation of the organization's media communication plan. However, for those emergencies that rise to that level, the designated spokesperson will be activated to coordinate with the media and relay information to them. It must be clear to all staff who that is and what the procedure is for referring requests for information to the

Case in Point
Information Technology Outage at Yale New Haven Health

Health care facilities' dependence on information technology (IT) for clinical and business applications means that IT outages present a broad array of challenges to the organizations where they occur. As electronic medical records (EMRs) become the norm, a greater proportion of internal communication is done via e-mail, and the whole host of business functions have been computerized, a broad IT outage—such as that experienced by Yale New Haven Health (New Haven, Connecticut) in 2014—has the potential to adversely affect patient care, as well as business continuity.

It is essential, therefore, to include IT outages in disaster planning. IT emergency planning, which, for many organizations, falls under the heading of business continuity planning (BCP), follows the same patterns as other kinds of emergency planning. Lessons learned during IT emergency events and drills can applied to other kinds of emergency planning and vice versa. In both cases, robust planning and clear processes for communication are keys to success.

Mitigation and Preparation

At Yale New Haven Health, Information Technology Services (ITS) operations are directed by a duty officer who is responsible for escalating incidents for possible declarations of disaster. During an incident, the duty officer compiles information from ITS staff, users, and vendor partners to inform his or her decision whether to escalate. If an incident causes or has the potential to cause an outage of more than four hours or to severely affect operations, then the duty officer will notify senior leadership. However, the duty officer need not wait until he or she has decided to recommend escalation to inform senior leaders, and indeed notifying senior leadership that there is a problem early on in the process allows leadership and other staff to begin to prepare for disaster operations or more limited changes in procedures. (*See* Figure 3-2 on page 48.)

The duty officer, when he or she contacts senior leadership, should be ready to provide detailed information of the problem or incident, including whether or not the cause has been determined, what steps have been taken to remedy the problem, whether ITS and its vendor partners have the resources to solve the problem, an estimate of how long it will take to implement a fix, and what systems or operations are likely to be affected. The senior leadership team can then make an informed decision as to whether a declaration of disaster should be made. In some cases, a more limited modification of operations will suffice while ITS fixes the problem. In other cases, downtime operations may be implemented in some departments but not in others.

In all cases, it is critical for senior leadership and ITS to know the maximum allowable downtime for each system under its control. This maximum allowable downtime is a function of how long the departments served by these systems can function effectively using downtime procedures, such as paper forms and non-networked computers. It is absolutely critical that staff are trained in the downtime procedures and know how to use the special downtime devices. Cloud storage can also be useful in enabling certain functions using computers that are not connected to the main organization network.

(continued on page 48)

The figure following illustrates Yale New Haven Health's decision-making and communications process for IT incidents.

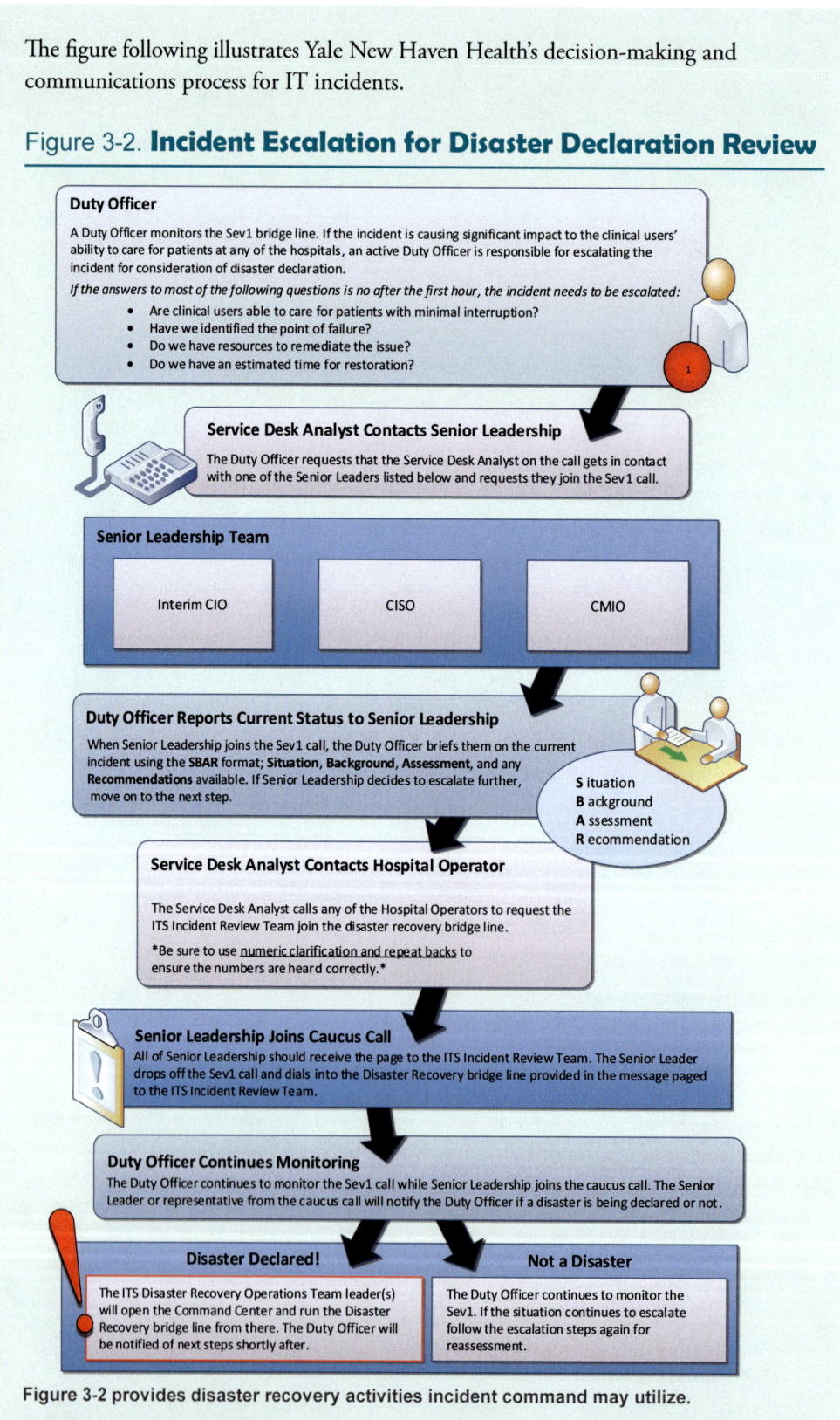

Figure 3-2. **Incident Escalation for Disaster Declaration Review**

Figure 3-2 provides disaster recovery activities incident command may utilize.

Source: Paturas JL. "Real-life health system network outage: Lessons learned." Presentation given at the Joint Commission Emergency Preparedness Conference, Lake Buena Vista, FL. May 1, 2015. Used with permission.

Response and Recovery

On July 11, 2014, at 10:00 a.m., ITS at Yale New Haven Health began receiving reports of connectivity problems from users. The ITS duty officer declared a Severity 1 situation, in which numerous individuals simultaneously experienced critical breakdowns in their technological systems. ITS staff quickly located the problem and determined that large portions of the network, including the EMR, were being rendered unusable. They engaged the assistance of the equipment vendor in diagnosing the problem and coming up with a remedy. Meanwhile, the duty officer informed senior leadership, who made the disaster declaration. Staff were informed via e-mail and paging to initiate downtime procedures. The equipment vendor was able to isolate the problem in less than an hour from the Severity 1 declaration. The affected device was removed from the network by 2:25 p.m., and users regained access to the EMR and were able to initiate recovery procedures by 2:45 p.m.

Assessment

Following the incident, after-action surveys were distributed across the entire Yale New Haven Health system to help senior leadership assess the system's response and make recommendations for improvement. These surveys were compiled into a comprehensive after-action report, which listed issues across The Joint Commission's six critical areas of disaster response and suggestions for improvement.

In general terms, the after-action report found that communication between ITS and senior leadership needed to start sooner. The disaster declaration needed to come sooner in the process. And procedures for notification and communication were inconsistent from site to site and department to department, leading to some sites not receiving notification or updates.

After-action surveys indicated that further training was needed for staff and various departments in downtime operations, as downtime response was inconsistent. Some departments lacked the proper paper forms. Some staff had difficulty locating or identifying downtime computer equipment. It is critical for every organization to know how to handle these situations by exercising annual drills or tabletop reviews.

Most importantly, the assessment team determined that criteria governing the decision to issue disaster declarations, initiate the EOP, and institute the Hospital Incident Command System (HICS) needed to be standardized to facilitate quick and informed decision making by senior leadership.

---

spokesperson. Organizations can establish a press office to operate as a central clearinghouse for information to be released to the public via the media, such as infection prevention information, first aid and treatment information, or updates on the health care organization's function or critical needs. This kind of communication will help keep the public informed, mitigate excessive requests for information, and ease confusion and concern. It may also allow hospitals to, for instance, appeal for blood donations, or direct well-meaning would-be donors to other locations in order to prevent the hospital being overwhelmed.

Capacity Builder

Emergency Telecommunications: Government Emergency Telecommunications Service (GETS)[1]

What Is It?

The Department of Homeland Security Office of Emergency Communications offers the GETS program to provide emergency preparedness teams with a communications resource that will grant them priority over other callers when using wireline networks in an emergency. The Wireless Priority Service (WPS) program gives its users priority when using cellular communications networks.

Who Should Use It?
- Police departments
- 9-1-1 call centers
- Emergency medical services (EMS)
- Health care organizations
- Public health and safety agencies

How Does It Work?

Health care and safety organizations enroll in the program and receive access cards and personal identification numbers (PINs). This program is available at all times; however, it is a critical resource during disasters and other crises. Organizations can exchange crucial information to coordinate response and recovery operations while bypassing the deluge of calls likely to inundate communications systems.

REFERENCE

1. Department of Homeland Security. *Government Emergency Telecommunications Service.* Accessed Jun 21, 2016. https://www.fcc.gov/general/government-emergency-telecommunications-service.

As with staff and external agencies, contact lists for local media outlets should be kept in the incident command center and shared communitywide. In addition, information can be made available to the public via social media. The PIO and press office staff may want to, as part of their emergency planning, work to develop an array of media advisory templates that can be updated and adapted to whatever emergencies arise. This way, the organization will have a preplanned information response to a number of emergency scenarios—whether it be an infectious disease outbreak, various kinds of natural disasters, an active shooter situation, or other emergency situations. Drills in relaying information and testing systems will prepare leaders and staff to communicate more effectively when it becomes necessary to convey details of a true crisis situation to those affected and the public at large.

Suppliers

Organizations must also communicate with vendors of essential supplies, equipment, and services, before and during an emergency. This requirement ties in with other emergency management standards that concern strategies for managing resources and assets during emergencies (*see* Chapter 4 for more detail), but it mainly emphasizes the need for communicating with those individuals and organizations that provide the resources necessary for the organization to operate. For example, the organization should identify in advance vendors who provide essential supplies such as medications, personal protective equipment, or linens, and services that range from utilities to contract employees.

> ## Community Collaboration
>
>
>
> ### Coordinating with the Media
> The media can be a helpful partner in emergency response and recovery. Help manage media relations during an emergency by answering the following questions during planning phases:
> - Has an area within the organization been designated for receiving the media—both inside and outside the facility?
> - Is the receiving area for the media located a sufficient distance from the emergency department or where patients are being treated, the command post, and waiting areas for relatives, family, and friends?
> - Does the area designated for the media have telephone, Wi-Fi, and television access?
> - Has a staff member(s) been designated to control and take care of the needs of the media?
> - Has a spokesperson for the organization been identified?
> - Do staff know how to route calls or inquiries from reporters?
> - Has the designated spokesperson been provided with a set of key messages approved by organization leadership?
> - Has a plan been created to guide the internal spokesperson's communications with emergency management agencies or other lead community agencies?
> - Are procedures in place for handling requests for information from the media and for updating that information?
> - Are procedures in place for responding to requests that are received after business hours from reporters?
> - Are procedures in place for responding to a reporter(s) who arrives at the facility?
> - Are plans in place for how the organization's website and/or social media pages can be used to disseminate information and for how that information will be updated on the website?

Communication regarding disaster inventories and procurement of resources takes place as part of ongoing planning and preparedness.

The health care organization must maintain listings of supplies, services, and equipment most critical to the type of emergency at the outset and for ongoing response operations, and maintain contact information for the primary suppliers and backup sources. A dynamic inventory control system could be used to track amount, location, and utilization of resources and assets throughout response and recovery; key personnel may keep backup reference lists for quick access in the event of technological disruptions. During response and recovery, the organization must periodically contact suppliers regarding any changing needs or to confirm its suppliers' ability to meet anticipated needs.

Other Health Care Organizations
No organization faces an emergency in a vacuum. Emergency conditions, the demand for resources, the need for additional staff, and other factors may affect health care organizations in the rest of the community, in neighboring communities, and throughout the region. Therefore, organizations must create plans for communicating with other nearby health care

organizations. In this way organizations can coordinate efforts to cope with patient surges, scarcity of resources, and other challenges.

As with other channels of communication, organizations must keep a list of organizations to be notified when the EOP is initiated, including the names and contact information of key leaders in those organizations and how best to contact them in an emergency. Information on the resources and capabilities of these organizations should be updated on an ongoing basis to maintain a current picture of the assistance they may provide or the resources they may need.

Organizations could maintain an updated list of organizations that provide similar services to their own and those that provide complementary or supplementary services. Emergency managers can then develop plans for resource sharing, evacuation procedures, and other contingency planning. Some of this activity can be coordinated through local departments of health under the auspices of the local or regional emergency operations center; this kind of coordination and information sharing is increasing through online systems that allow coalition members to update their own information and see that of other members in real time.

Alternative Care Sites

Finally, organizations must identify alternative care sites that meet the needs of their patients as part of their EOP, and a contact list for those sites is maintained in the incident command center, with redundant hard or digital copies kept separately as needed.

It is important to consider how the organization will maintain communication with alternative care sites during an emergency. The challenges will vary depending on the site. Some sites will have relatively robust communication systems already in place, but if, for instance, patients are relocated to sites that are not health care facilities, there must be a plan for establishing and maintaining communication with those sites. Cell phones, two-way radios, satellite phones, or ham radios may provide the needed lines of contact.

It is up to each organization to identify its needs, according to the capabilities of its identified alternative care sites, and to acquire the necessary equipment and train their personnel in its use. Organizations should keep in mind their plans for an internal surge as well.

Backup Communication Systems

When an emergency occurs, telephones and cell phones often fail and leave organizations without their usual means of communication. A contingency plan for backup of internal and external communication systems is crucial to ensuring that organizations can still communicate even in the face of the unexpected.

Primary and Secondary Options

Phone line options include maintaining a backup power source for internal phone switches, diversifying existing phone lines, and planning for the prioritized repair of existing phone lines. In addition, organizations may consider using satellite phones during emergencies, as these phones communicate using signals that are beamed to and from satellites, enabling them to continue to function when a natural disaster has damaged landlines or wireless telephone infrastructure. Alternative communication equipment options include the following:

Radio Equipment	Wire Line	Combination
Two-way radios	Telephone	Smart phones
Pagers	Fax machine	Satellite phones
Broadcast radio	Computer modem	
Television	Public address system	
Satellite	Organization intercom	
Ham radios and local police, fire, and EMS radios		
Direct line to county Emergency Operations Center		

Communications options aside from the telephone include the use of a public address system or closed-circuit television system. Organizations might also use an alarm system that signifies when the facility is in an emergency-response mode. Any of these options could be followed up with messages on the organization's website and social media pages, as well as e-mails to all staff and employees.

Other methods for communication include wireless e-mail devices, 800 MHz radios, ham radios, and walkie-talkies. Some organizations opt for satellite TV during hurricane season in case cable goes out and they need to stay informed of impending weather conditions.

Equipment Maintenance

A regular routine of equipment maintenance for emergency equipment is essential for reliable performance and rapid repairs to help get the facility back on the communication track following an emergency. Because radio and microwave systems can be damaged, organizations should have available replacement supplies of antennas, coaxial cable, and other hardware susceptible to damage. They need to verify through inspections that telephone lines coming into the communication center are buried, clearly marked, and protected from possible damage. They will also need to stockpile extra batteries for any battery-operated equipment on site, and to create a maintenance schedule to test and replace depleted batteries. An emergency situation may escalate or evolve over time, so preparing for primary system failure is a critical area of emergency planning.

IN SUMMARY

- The EOP should outline how information is to be communicated internally and externally. Staff should be trained in these procedures, including how to address primary, and even secondary, communication systems failure.
- Up-to-date contact information for staff, community partners, vendors, alternative care sites, and any other critical contacts should be kept in the incident command center and updated regularly.
- Technology is used to facilitate communication and build redundant systems.

CHAPTER 4

Managing Resources and Assets

STANDARDS FOCUS

EM.02.01.01 The organization has an Emergency Operations Plan.

EM.02.02.03 As part of its Emergency Operations Plan, the organization prepares for how it will manage resources and assets during emergencies.

AT A GLANCE

- Obtaining and replenishing resources
- Planning for patient surge
- Managing resources during evacuations

WHO IS INVOLVED?

- Procurement or purchasing department leadership
- Clinical and engineering leaders
- Vendors and suppliers
- Emergency manager
- Coalition partners
- Departments of health and other government agencies

Why Is This Critical?

To ensure an effective response to an emergency, organizations must consider what items will be needed to adequately care for patients. In the event that an organization's community is affected by a disaster and cannot provide resources to the health care organization, plans must take into account the risk that some assets might not be available. For instance, a disruption to or contamination of the water supply would not only prevent access to clean drinking water, it has the potential to create a number of other problems, including loss of the ability to sterilize equipment, loss of fire-suppression capability, loss of sanitation services, loss of decontamination capability, and so forth. It is essential that organization leaders know what resources and assets are available to them in an emergency and have plans for how to manage scarce resources, replenish them when possible, and track usage and consumption as the situation evolves.

Key Planning Concepts for Resources and Assets

Under ordinary circumstances, health care organizations replenish supplies and resources routinely to acquire all they need for safe, high-quality patient care. An emergency will likely cause increased demand for limited resources and assets. Such a situation may stress vendor inventories, resulting in organizations being unable to acquire sufficient quantities of supplies to address patient needs.

Obtaining and Replenishing Supplies

Organizations must identify supplies they will need in an emergency and make an inventory of what they have on hand. Supply needs will vary with the type and duration of the emergency, but organizations can use the hazard vulnerability analysis (HVA; described in Chapter 2) to identify likely needs and to help determine adequate supply levels for those items. After taking inventory of their current resources and assets, emergency management staff will need to consider their budgets and plan for how they will allocate funds for obtaining and/or replenishing resources to meet the needs of an emergency situation. (*See* Figure 4-1 below for a sample budgeting form that may be used as a way for organizations to identify the expense needs for emergency requirements.) It is crucial that organizations have plans in place to allocate their financial resources to meet their emergency needs.

Figure 4-1. Disaster Preparedness Budget

Catastrophe/Disaster Preparedness Budget							
Department:	Administration						
	DEPARTMENTAL PROGRAM						
Expense Category	Staying Up to Date	Emergency Management Coordinator	Command Center Space	Security	Training and Drills	Risk Management	Total All Programs
Operating expenses:				All depts			
Salaries and wages	$ –	$ 50,000	$ –	$ –	$ 250,000	$ –	$ 300,000
Payroll taxes and benefits	$ –	$ 14,000	$ –	$ –	$ 62,500	$ –	$ 76,500
Contract services	$ –	$ –	$ –	$ 350,000	$ 5,000	$ –	$ 355,000
Education and travel	$ 12,000	$ 3,000	$ –	$ –	$ –	$ –	$ 15,000
Space costs	$ –	$ 6,000	$ –	$ –	$ –	$ –	$ 6,000
Utilities	$ –	$ 800	$ 3,600	$ –	$ –	$ –	$ 4,400
Communications	$ –	$ 500	$ 2,500	$ –	$ –	$ –	$ 3,000
Commodities and supplies	$ –	$ 1,000	$ 1,000	$ –	$ –	$ –	$ 2,000
Insurance	$ –	$ –	$ –	$ –	$ –	$ 350,000	$ 350,000
Leases and rentals	$ –	$ –	$ –	$ –	$ –	$ –	$ –
Depreciation	$ –	$ –	$ 12,000	$ –	$ –	$ –	$ 12,000
Other	$ –	$ –	$ –	$ –	$ –	$ –	$ –
TOTAL IN OPERATING EXPENSES	$ 12,000	$ 75,300	$ 19,100	$ 350,000	$ 317,500	$ 350,000	$1,123,900
Capital purchases	$ –	$ –	$ 3,000	$ –	$ –	$ –	$ 3,000
TOTAL CASH BUDGET	$ 12,000	$ 75,300	$ 22,100	$ 350,000	$ 317,500	$ 350,000	$1,126,900
Sources of funds:							
General hospital revenues	$ 12,000	$ 75,300	$ 19,100	$ 350,000	$ 317,000	$ 350,000	$1,123,900
Grants	$ –	$ –	$ 3,000	$ –	$ –	$ –	$ 3,000
Borrowing	$ –	$ –	$ –	$ –	$ –	$ –	$ 76,500
Other	$ –	$ –	$ –	$ –	$ –	$ –	$ 76,500
Total sources of funds	$ 12,000	$ 75,300	$ 22,100	$ 350,000	$ 317,500	$ 350,000	$1,126,900
Budget over (under) funded	$ –	$ –	$ –	$ –	$ –	$ –	$ –

To Summary

Figure 4-1 is designed to help health care leaders create a financial plan as part of their emergency preparedness activities.

Source: Centers for Disease Control and Prevention. Hospital Disaster Preparedness Budget Model. Tucker E. 2014. Accessed Jun 22, 2016. www.cdc.gov/phpr/healthcare/documents/Disaster_Budget_Model.xlsx.

Medications

The Emergency Operations Plan (EOP) must consider what kinds of medications may be needed in certain emergency situations. Likely they will need to replenish depleted stocks of medicine that might be easy to find during normal operations but become scarce in unusual circumstances. When planning for emergencies, emergency managers might consider a number of possible sources for critical medications, including but not limited to the following:

- Supplies the organization has on hand
- Strategic caches the organization has set aside specifically for emergencies
- Supplementary supplies delivered through surge agreements with vendors
- Supplies secured through agreements with local pharmacies
- Supplies available from other facilities operated by a parent company
- Government supplies
- Health care coalition or community supplies

Certain crisis situations—such as infectious disease outbreaks or exposure to hazardous and toxic materials—might require a much-needed antidote or a quick-acting remedy available only in rationed supplies (if at all). In such situations, and in major disasters that overwhelm or threaten to overwhelm local and regional health systems, medication may be made available through the Centers for Disease Control and Prevention (CDC) Strategic National Stockpile (SNS). Through the SNS, for example, the CDC can rapidly deploy antibiotics and other medications to combat emerging influenza outbreaks. Similarly, the CDC's Chemical Hazards Emergency Medical Management (CHEMM) program provides significant quantities of antidote in the event of a chemical attack or release. Almost 2,000 CHEMPACKs are already strategically placed at hospitals and fire stations across the nation, so immediate access is supported.

Although it is difficult for organizations to foresee the particular medication needs that might become necessary only in extraordinary situations, they must have plans to work with outside organizations to obtain less common antidotes and remedies. An umbrella plan can be adjusted according to the nature of the emergency. Emergency management teams should partner with their pharmacy and procurement leaders to research the availability of medication and the logistics for acquiring it—both the common and the rare medications.

In any case, as in other areas, solid mitigation and preparation activities are the foundation of medication resource management for disasters. Hospital managers and emergency managers must be able to determine with specificity the inventory and track the use of essential medications. Procurement professionals can work in advance of an emergency to streamline the supply chain. Consolidating procurement to a smaller number of vendors simplifies procurement in an emergency and leaves other vendors as alternate options if supplies get tight or delivery becomes problematic. In addition, larger vendors may have multiple warehouses and thus be better equipped to deliver during an emergency. It is also critical to understand the medication inventories of other health care coalition providers. In a large event, the health care coalition may have to rally around community resources before external resources become available.

> ### Setting Spotlight
>
> **Nursing Care Center**
> In the first hours after the September 11, 2001, attacks on the World Trade Center, the staff of St. Margaret's Home, a nursing care center located six blocks from Ground Zero, inventoried every department's supplies because they knew that there were not going to be normal deliveries the next day. In fact, although the State Department of Public Health began sending supplies, St. Margaret's had trouble getting them. No vehicles were moving, and the supplies were being held up at the police checkpoints/incident command post. The organization's executive director rode his bike to the post to get the supplies released. In another instance, he rode his bike to meet the milk delivery truck and escort it back through police lines to his facility. The executive director faxed letters of entry for the vendors, giving the incident command post detailed information, including a physical description of the vendor.

Capacity Builder

Training Staff to Use Strategic National Stockpile Ventilators

Many hospitals are equipped with lifesaving mechanical ventilators designed to manage respiratory failure brought on by illness or injury. But these large and expensive devices are not found in ample supply at health care facilities across the country. Fortunately, the Centers for Disease Control and Prevention's (CDC) Strategic National Stockpile (SNS) has a repository of thousands of compact, portable, and battery-powered ventilators, available in three different models, that can be dispatched to the affected area upon request.

Respiratory therapists, acute care nurses, physicians, and other hospital clinicians responsible for managing ventilators are skilled at using the devices provided in their facilities. However, they may lack the training needed to operate an SNS ventilator. This limitation could become particularly crucial during a large-scale public health emergency (PHE), when fast and efficient response is needed to save lives.

Consequently, it's important for leaders to ensure that their staff receive the education and training needed to use this specialized equipment and to incorporate this training into their disaster management and emergency operations planning. In fact, SNS ventilator training should be part of the Emergency Operations Plan. Staff should know how to respond to an influx of potentially infectious patients based on many scenarios identified in the hazard vulnerability analysis, including a PHE resulting in many patients requiring ventilators, and how to contact resources to request additional ventilators.

The CDC partnered with the American Association for Respiratory Care (AARC) to provide online training resources, including videos and manuals on SNS ventilators (http://aarc.org/resources/sns_vent_training).

Identifying the Target Audience

It's crucial to provide standardized training of all medical personnel expected to have ventilator-associated responsibilities. Both standardized pre-event training (coordinated training of medical personnel before a PHE) and just-in-time training (trainings conducted during a PHE) have been identified within the Department of Health and Human Services (HHS) Public Health Emergency Medical Countermeasures Enterprise disaster preparedness framework as appropriate models to increase the number of medical personnel who can manage patients on SNS mechanical ventilators.

Although certain staff may have proficiency with ventilators in general, each of the three models within the SNS has different features, capabilities, and operating instructions for such functions as powering on and adjusting settings and alarms. Proper training is required to do the following:
- Know the devices' capabilities and limitations
- Make certain that the devices are set up and used properly
- Troubleshoot devices quickly when something goes wrong

Proper training will ensure that providers assign the right ventilator to the right patients. Professionals need to know when these devices are sufficient to manage victims of the event or when to use the basic modes provided by these devices for less ill patients who are not direct victims, such as those suffering postoperative respiratory failure.

Emergency Readiness Tools

Although it's reassuring to know that SNS ventilator training materials are now available to anyone anytime on the AARC's website, health care facility administrators must be proactive and ensure that their clinical professionals know about these resources and utilize them to receive the necessary training, per Joint Commission Emergency Management (EM) and Infection Control and Prevention (IC) requirements. Emergency managers can build related scenarios into their twice-a-year drills—such as a respiratory emergency scenario like a pandemic flu that involves the use of ventilators.

Health care organizations can adapt the ARRC's online materials to meet the emergency preparedness training needs of their staff, such as developing train-the-trainer presentations, continuing education offerings, and question-and-answer sessions. Employers can also attend additional instructional opportunities, such as hands-on workshops where attendees can touch, test, and interact with SNS ventilators. In the future, SNS ventilator training may be available at professional organization conferences or ventilator manufacturers.

Health care organizations also need to know how to access ventilators from the SNS in a crisis. The steps involved in such a dispatch include the following:

1. Local officials determine the need for additional resources and request assistance through their emergency management agency or health department.
2. Upon receipt of the request, HHS and the CDC evaluate the situation and determine the appropriate response strategy.
3. After SNS delivers the ventilators to specified receiving sites, the state or other receiving entity distributes the ventilators from those sites to medical treatment facilities, based on the individual states' "receive, stage, and store" plan for distribution of any SNS assets.

To date, SNS ventilators have never actually been used during a PHE, although they have been forward-deployed and stored nearby for several events. For more information, go to http://www.cdc.gov/phpr/stockpile/stockpile.htm.

Community Collaboration

Resource-Sharing Questions

- What resources and assets (supplies, beds, staff, and so forth) might be shared in a regional or prolonged disaster?
- What could our organization provide?
- What might our organization need from other organizations?
- What provisions can we make to share or obtain resources and assets with health care organizations within our community during a prolonged emergency?
- What provisions can we make to share or obtain resources and assets with health care organizations outside our area during a prolonged emergency?

Medical Supplies

Regular review of medical supplies is an important component of planning for emergency situations. Organizations should determine current supplies such as ventilators (adult, pediatric, neonate, and other), intravenous (IV) pumps, IV poles, oxygen cardiac monitors, blankets, suction machines, beds, stretchers, and wheelchairs, as well as personal protective equipment such as masks, gloves, eye protection, and face shields. Rotation of certain supplies is important to maintain their viability. Through continual training simulations, staff and leadership can learn to assess the limitations of their stock and understand how to supplement their supplies should extenuating circumstances require it.

The HVA should be used as a guide to identify events that may require additional medical and other supplies. Supply needs will differ according to specific circumstances. Exercises covering the most likely and the most resource-intensive emergency scenarios can help managers determine what their likely resource needs will be and how to meet them efficiently. In the event that numerous organizations require the same resource at the same time—for example, an N95 respirator during an outbreak of the H1N1 influenza—organizations may need to consider alternative equipment sources during development of the EOP.

Setting Spotlight

Home Care

Caring for patients in their homes presents certain challenges in emergency management. Although a home care agency's Emergency Operations Plan (EOP) addresses the same critical areas as other health care organizations, it takes a different approach in managing those needs in a home environment.

One of the most important resources to be managed by home care agencies during an emergency is transportation assistance and priority access to fuel. Due to the nature of home care, staff must travel to monitor and care for patients in their homes. These care settings may be located across a broad area, which makes it critical for home care providers to maintain solid access to transportation, possibly through agreements with suppliers.

An agency's EOP may plan for this access with a number of community agencies—such as police, law enforcement, fire departments, and the local health department. The agency might document arrangements with local vendors, such as bus companies that supply buses for schools. The agency might also contract with private ambulance or even taxi companies. Whatever means of transport assistance providers are able to attain, they will also need backup contingencies. A regional emergency might stress the availability of transportation, should it be required by multiple sources at once. Transport may even prove to be inoperable, due to impassable roads or scarcity of gas. Agencies will need to provide their staff with alternative maps if their usual routes are compromised.

In some instances, assuming it is still possible for patients to remain in their homes, home care staff will need to prioritize the individual needs of their patients and their personal safety and security. Regularly updated medical records make it possible for providers to determine which patients would experience the most adverse effects due to interruption of care—such as those relying on life-sustaining medication and equipment—and make every effort to reach them first. Patients who will remain stable if treatment is temporarily suspended will be prioritized next. Patients able to treat themselves or with assistance until services resume would receive final priority. Decisions such as these are difficult to make, but they must be taken into account when developing the EOP. Communitywide exercises make it possible to identify and mitigate vulnerabilities.

Source: Home Care Association of New York State; New York State Health Care Providers. Primer on Home Care Emergency Preparedness in New York State. 2015. Accessed Jun 22, 2016. http://www.hca-nys.org/documents/HomeCareEPPrimer.pdf.

When preparing caches of emergency supplies, the emergency team must plan for a number of patient populations. Pediatric casualties will require proper-sized equipment and specially sized dosages of medications, for instance—on hand or stored where they can be retrieved easily. The team must also consider the needs of other vulnerable populations such as bariatric, elderly, or special needs patients, or those with serious chronic conditions (for example, dialysis, cardiac, cancer), or addictions or mental illness. It is important to stockpile and track emergency equipment and equipment for special populations, to provide for its regular maintenance, and to provide staff with periodic training needed to maintain competency in its use.

Preparedness teams will store many of their material needs on site. In consideration of space constraints and for security of resources, it will be necessary to keep caches of some supplies off site. The EOP will identify how these critical supplies will be made available when they

> ### Capacity Builder
>
> Although organizations should have on hand supplies for the most likely emergencies, as identified by the hazard vulnerability analysis, common additional supplies needed in an emergency situation include the following:
>
> - Meals ready to eat (MREs)
> - Stretchers
> - Intravenous supplies
> - Oxygen
> - Cardiac monitors
> - Blankets
> - Pharmaceuticals, including narcotics
> - Orthopedic software and plastering
> - Ventilators (adult, pediatric, neonate, and so forth)
> - Intravenous (IV) pumps
> - IV poles
> - Suction machines
> - Beds
> - Wheelchairs
> - Personal protective equipment (PPE)
> - Masks, including powered air purifying respirators (PAPR)
> - Gloves
> - Eye protection
> - Face shields
>
> As with any stockpiled equipment, these items not only need to be obtained, but also maintained to protect against expired batteries, corrosion, and other effects of long-term storage.

are required at the location of patient care, whether it be at the organization's facility or in an alternative care site.

Nonmedical Supplies

Additional medical equipment and supplies may be required, either by an influx of patients or because these items are requested through health care coalition partnerships. Emergency stockpiles of nonmedical supplies, such as food, water, and fuel, should be first assessed to understand organizational needs. A plan must then be developed to ensure there is access to a 96-hour supply. Additional supplies may be obtained and maintained in case the organization is temporarily unable to replenish these supplies through normal means. In some instances, such as in the event of a slowly developing weather emergency, health care organizations can request for and receive large reserves of essential supplies to withstand its effects. However, these supply reserves must be planned in advance of the situation that requires them. Surge agreements and memoranda of understanding may be useful in facilitating this process.

The organization's preparedness team should partner with procurement to work with vendors and suppliers along with community agencies to create preplanned supply surges. In the

Vulnerable Populations

Managing Space for Long Term Care Populations

In long term care settings, whether they be in behavioral health care facilities, nursing care centers, or home care and hospice locations, the emphasis on disaster management is on the population served if it is an internal disaster. Every long term health care setting must be prepared to effectively shelter in place, or to have preestablished relationships with other local long term care organizations to move residents from one facility to another or, in the event of a community disaster, to safely transport residents to locations farther away. It could also mean that care is provided at alternative sites that might have austere care environments. This requires a systematic and redundant plan that takes into account individual needs, such as ensuring that patients' medication regimen is not disrupted in an emergency evacuation or that sensory aids such as eyeglasses, hearing aids, and so forth, are accounted for.

Effective emergency management also depends on strong relationships among health care organizations and the community at large. Regional partnerships must be built and maintained to integrate planned responses before an emergency or a disaster occurs. This is particularly important when the emergency involves a special population such as the vulnerable elderly. In the case of a communitywide emergency, all health care organizations might be needed—to assist with triage and urgent care of victims, provide nonurgent care to others, shelter community members or patients from facilities that have been evacuated, or supply specific staff and/or supplies to other organizations.

It is critical to have conversations with hospitals to ascertain the ability of the organization to absorb long term care patients. Hospitals have finite staffing and bed resources and may be severely limited in their ability to continue meeting community needs if all available beds are taken. The role of the hospital should be to treat patients who have a medical need, not housing.

event that the emergency manager initiates the EOP, all parties should be clear on the expectations of the plan. Key suppliers would deliver predetermined quantities of specified items, and the health care team and community partners would be responsible for maintaining, distributing, and using them. It is a good idea to periodically test key suppliers to see how the supplies will be delivered and how long it would take for delivery.

Space

Emergency planners should also consider space as a key asset and plan for its management in an emergency. If an emergency is predicted to cause a sudden influx of patients in the emergency department (ED), organizations may want to plan for the expedited admission of patients already there, perhaps also moving the most stable patients in the facility to alternative care sites, in case of a mass-casualty event. If there is an infectious disease outbreak event, a radiological event, or other event leading to a rapid influx, a plan needs to be in place to create sufficient space to isolate and treat or decontaminate the resulting incoming patients. Patient surge due to mass-casualty events can rapidly cause an increase in patient load in the ED. Efficient throughput of patients to keep the ED population low, under normal operations, is an operational goal that can help underpin emergency response.

Because many organizations and community health care systems operate near 100% capacity, emergency planners may want to consider one or more of the following strategies to deal with a major or prolonged patient surge:
- Tapping coalition partners to alleviate surge
- Converting outpatient treatment spaces for extended patient care
- Creating alternative care spaces within existing facilities (hallways, conference rooms, and so forth)
- Opening closed/shuttered sections of the organization
- Using designated alternative care sites
- Deploying temporary health care facilities through the community's incident command structure and the federal disaster system

Some emergencies will require staff to remain at the facility for an extended period—for example, during major snowfalls or hurricanes. Organizations will need to plan ahead of time for respite space where staff can sleep, shower, and unwind during downtime.

Sharing Resources

Organizations should include in their EOPs potential sharing of resources and assets with health care coalitions within and outside the community. In a regional or prolonged disaster, several organizations in one region may use the same vendors for common supplies such as linens, medications, and fuel. If the emergency is severe and long lasting, multiple organizations relying on the same vendors could exhaust available equipment and supplies inventories. Therefore, having relationships with suppliers outside of the organization's region is smart planning. Some organizations might find it easier to negotiate with local or national health care associations to develop shared vendor-purchasing agreements in emergencies. In addition, both health care organizations and vendors should have their own backups in place. Setting up credit lines before an emergency is much easier to do as part of the emergency planning process rather than trying to do it during the emergency.

In addition to sharing resources through vendor arrangements, organizations that are part of health care systems often share resources available through their parent organizations or sister facilities in other communities, regions, or states. The development of local or regional hospital or health care coalitions can be a great help in coordinating resource management efforts. Participating in a coalition can provide preexisting relationships through which resources can be shared among the members in the event of a communitywide disaster response, when large quantities of supplies and equipment may be needed off site (for example, earthquake response, transit accidents, or other mass-casualty events). Coalition partners can work together to help ensure that patients across the community can be provided the right care at the right time from the right level of health care provider.

Evacuation-Related Issues

Providing for patient safety and essential medical care during evacuation is of paramount importance in the decision to evacuate. A patient may be en route for a very short period of time, but in cases of communitywide disasters, a patient may be en route for hours. The resources and assets that travel with every patient during evacuation—including accompanying staff—must be carefully considered and provided; taking an advance inventory of resources during evacuation is important. Organizations should consider the acuity and age of the patient during transfer, as some patients may require a significant amount of equipment and staff. For example, a neonatal intensive care unit patient may require four staff members, multiple pumps and monitors, and an incubator for transfer.

Many supplies will be consumed en route, but equipment will return to the original organization. It is important to track ventilators, IV pumps, stretchers, wheelchairs, and so forth so that when emergency operations are terminated all resources can be accounted for and equipment can be restored to its proper locations as quickly as possible as part of the recovery phase.

How patients are transported in the event of evacuation must also be considered in emergency management planning and arranged with the transport service in advance. In some cases the hospital or other health care organization will have appropriate transport vehicles in its fleet. In other cases the transportation will be arranged with private ambulance services, emergency medical services (EMS), or through other means. Communication with police or fire services is important to ensure that evacuation routes are clear so that the patient does not encounter unanticipated delays.

Creating plans, policies, and procedures to govern patient transfers will help mitigate confusion and facilitate uninterrupted patient care throughout the evacuation. This is another area in which participating in coalitions can be of great help. Protocols for transfer of evacuated patients are essential and should be shared in advance of evacuation—this includes direct conversation and confirmation with the receiving sites before patients are moved.

IN SUMMARY

- Stockpile caches of critical supplies for use during emergencies.
- Coordinate emergency procedures with key vendors and suppliers to ensure that needed supplies can be replenished during an emergency.
- Look to health care coalitions for good tools and strategies to plan for resource scarcity and communitywide disaster response.
- Manage space as a resource during and after emergencies.
- Plan to have the resources on hand that will be needed during an evacuation.

CHAPTER 5

Ensuring Safety and Security

STANDARDS FOCUS

EM.02.01.01 The organization has an Emergency Operations Plan.

EM.02.02.05 As part of its Emergency Operations Plan, the organization prepares for how it will manage security and safety during an emergency.

AT A GLANCE

- Coordinating with external security agencies
- Maintaining internal security
- Decontaminating patients
- Managing hazardous materials

WHO IS INVOLVED?

- Organization leadership
- Chief of security
- Safety officer
- Infection control chief
- Director of facilities management
- Director of behavioral health
- Director of social work
- Vendors and suppliers

Why Is This Critical?

Ensuring the safety and security of patients, staff, and other individuals within hospitals and other health care facilities is a primary responsibility of the organization. Every organization's mission is to deliver health care services to its community. Failure to protect those in the care of the organization from accidental harm (safety failure) or intentional harm (security failure) obviously runs counter to that mission, increasing the demand for services while simultaneously diminishing the organization's ability to provide them.

Key Planning Concepts for Safety and Security

Safety and security of patients and staff are primary responsibilities of the organization. Security within the organization and its facilities is critical to its ability to maintain crucial medical and behavioral health care services to patients. While safety and security are issues that should occupy emergency managers and organization leaders, all staff have a responsibility to be alert to possible threats. Staff require training in how to recognize threats to safety and security early. It is through the staff that the organization becomes aware of problems. Staff are the most familiar with what is normal and what is out of the ordinary in their workplace, which with training makes them a critical security asset to the organization.

Maintaining Internal Security

During an emergency, security staff should be present to facilitate access to key emergency response areas (for example, patient/family access to emergency flu clinic or parking lot triage tent) and to prevent unauthorized or agitated individuals or even groups of individuals from compromising the operations of the organization's emergency response. As part of emergency management planning, organizations must determine what types of safety and security issues are likely to arise and affect organization operations.

65

Authorized Access

To maintain internal security without substantially diminishing the organization's ability to function, emergency planners need to develop a plan for how to control who comes into and out of the facility and what areas of the building they are allowed to access. This planning needs to cover the movements of staff, patients, family members, contractors, vendors, local security personnel, maintenance and utility workers, and volunteers.

Monitoring Entrances

Preventing bottlenecks at points of entry during a major disaster may be difficult with an influx of patients and/or a large number of first responders, staff, or volunteers arriving in a short period of time. Extra security should be deployed in the emergency department (ED) and designated entrances for patients, visitors, and staff to ensure that unauthorized individuals (for example, the media) do not enter sensitive areas of the facility. Designating one or two access points for staff to enter the facility or to pass through an external security perimeter, and posting security at these points with staff lists to help them verify identities, can help staff enter the building throughout the response and recovery phases of an emergency, even if they happen not to have their official staff identification with them. The issuing of temporary generic staff badges or laminates may be a good way to bring staff into the facility quickly and identify their access privileges within the building.

Limiting Facility Sections

Within the facility, organizations may want to limit access to specific areas. Certainly, any area that has sustained physical damage should be closed to visitors, and probably to anyone not involved in repair and maintenance activities. Internal manned security checkpoints, key card access doors, cameras, and regular keyed locks can help limit access to sensitive areas; protect equipment, medications, and other supplies from damage, tampering, or theft; and control the movement of unauthorized individuals. It is imperative that the organization has a plan in place detailing which areas should be locked down in an emergency.

Managing Disruptive Behavior

During an event, it will not be unusual for patients, visitors, and staff to be under significant duress. Staff should be trained to identify and respond to escalating behavior. The emergency management team should work with representatives in behavioral health, social work, and clinical leadership to develop a team to respond to disruptive behavior. The team should be an active participant in emergency management drills. In smaller organizations, building a relationship with law enforcement may be critical for a timely response.

Controlling Transportation

The organization needs to plan to control and direct vehicular access to the facility. Dozens of vehicles, helicopters, and media converging on a health care organization can limit the ability of ambulances and other emergency transportation assets to reach their destinations, or to leave. Organizations may want to institute standing rules limiting or prohibiting vehicular access to the facility by staff and the general public during emergency response. Temporary signage can help direct nonessential traffic away from critical access points. And emergency medical services (EMS) can be informed by radio of changes to normal traffic flow and

Case in Point
Active Shooter Incident at Health First–Palm Bay Hospital

Health First–Palm Bay Hospital is a full-service 152-bed hospital located on Florida's Atlantic coast with a 22-bed emergency department serving more than 38,000 patients annually. On November 4, 2010, the facility was the site of an active shooter incident that lasted between three and four hours. Only a month before, James Kendig, then vice president for Safety and Security at the hospital, had published and distributed a quick reference guide to active shooter incident procedures The guide contained tips on how to recognize an active shooter, how to identify the signs of instability in coworkers, what information to convey to security personnel or law enforcement, and how to behave when law enforcement arrives.

Incident and Response

Shortly after a dispute with his landlord over the rent, an armed man entered the hospital and barricaded himself in the kitchen manager's office. Code Silver (active shooter) was declared, and law enforcement was alerted. Four local law enforcement agencies responded. Police surrounded the subject and attempted to persuade him to surrender. After three and a half hours, a police robot was deployed and found the subject dead of a self-inflicted gunshot wound.

Assessment and Conclusions

A postincident review was conducted with law enforcement. The review identified several areas of suboptimal response, and made recommendations for changes.

Problems identified included the following:
- There was a lack of access badges for law enforcement, who were forced to use the badges of staff.
- The incident command center was not activated.
- Law enforcement did not have access to hospital plans.
- Staff continued to enter the building during the standoff despite ongoing danger.
- The hospital disaster hotline was not used.
- There was no remote shutoff valve for natural gas.

Steps taken to improve future response included the following:
- Each of the four hospitals in the Health First network placed a "go kit" for law enforcement in their command centers. The "go kits" contain 20 access badges for law enforcement and hard copies of the hospitals' life safety drawings.
- Each of the four hospitals provided a thumb drive containing their life safety plans to local law enforcement.
- A yellow light was added above the employee entrance to warn staff not to enter in the event of an ongoing security situation.

Security staff leadership increased their coordination with local law enforcement, including attending meetings of local police leadership.

>
> ## Setting Spotlight
>
> ### Laboratory
>
> With the increased concern regarding possible use of biological, chemical, and radioactive materials as terrorism agents, a laboratory's Emergency Operations Plan (EOP) needs to consider a number of safety and security threats:
>
> - Employee screening
> - Personnel safety
> - Authorized access
> - Technology security
> - Containment of pathogens and toxins
> - Safe handling of specimens
>
> Employee screening is the front line of security. People working with potentially harmful substances must be trusted to do so with safety and integrity. They might be required by a laboratory to undergo a number of security checks not usually required by health care organizations and must meet the criteria of a number of regulating bodies.
>
> Personnel safety must be one of the top priorities in the EOP. Plans will include rigorous training for staff. Exercises on how to handle emergencies in the laboratory, such as the compromise of sensitive electronic information or the hazards of containing exposure to contaminants, need to be conducted on a regular basis.
>
> Facility safety and security are of paramount importance. The EOP must plan for the storage of essential supplies and critical agents such as toxins with the most stringent measures in mind. Access to these areas must be authorized and scrutinized by leaders. Emergency circumstances will put these accommodations to the test. The EOP needs to create a plan adaptable enough to withstand numerous and varied emergency scenarios.
>
> Should the containment of pathogens or other substances be compromised in any way, safety protocols must be in place to contain their impact and keep staff safe. Exposure to them should be as limited as possible—such as in the instance of physical damage to the facility or cleanup of the agents after the emergency has subsided.
>
> The EOP will need to address the handling, storage, and transportation of harmful substances—either within or outside the laboratory. Laboratory criteria, as well as state and/or government regulations, will determine these safety protocols.
>
> Overall, a laboratory's emergency management measures will offer the best line of defense against compounding the overall impact of an emergency situation.
>
> **Source:** Richmond JY, Nesby-O'Dell SL; Centers for Disease Control and Prevention. Laboratory security and emergency response guidance for laboratories working with select agents. MMWR Recomm Rep. 2002 Dec 6;51(RR-19):1–6. Accessed Jun 22, 2016. http://www.cdc.gov/mmwr/preview/mmwrhtml/rr5119a1.htm.

procedures. Security staff should be able to answer the following questions, based on prior planning in the Emergency Operations Plan (EOP):

- Do you have cones and other barriers to control sensitive traffic and parking areas?
- Do you have the personnel available for a quickly developing event to staff these areas?
- Do you have an agreement with local law enforcement or, if the event is in the same locale, other law enforcement (state or county or other municipal agencies) not involved in the emergency or disaster event?
- Do you have a plan to deal with the media? Where should they be staged?

In addition, facilities with helipads will need to coordinate their own staff with those at partner facilities and the public aviation authority to manage sending and receiving of patients, staff, and equipment via air.

Crowd Control

Among the greatest challenges to internal safety and security is controlling the movement of people already inside the building. Organizations may decide to set up one or more public access points at which people may be directed to the proper locations within the facility (such as family waiting rooms especially set up to provide information and support to families affected by the emergency).

If a crowd does form, the first step in gaining control is to establish a perimeter. Security personnel can also help to prevent crowds from forming by having clear information about how and where to direct patients and members of the community who might seek food or shelter from health care organizations during a disaster. Concentric rings of internal security will assist in limiting unauthorized access to security-sensitive areas.

Active Shooter Situations

The frequency of mass shooting events makes planning for active shooter situations a critical part of emergency planning, and health care facilities are no different. Emergency planners should work with security staff and local law enforcement agencies to devise a comprehensive plan for how the organization will respond to this scenario. The allowance or prohibition of firearms within the facility will necessarily affect response plans, as will the expectations and active shooter planning of local law enforcement agencies.

Staff training prior to a situation in how to recognize erratic or escalating behaviors before they reach a critical point is essential and can help staff defuse conflicts before they become emergencies. However, it is critical for staff across all departments to have and be familiar with active shooter response plans to take action for their safety and the safety of those around them. Staff training in active shooter response is essential, as it in some ways deviates from the usual staff response to potential patient risk and to the arrival of law enforcement. Patient care in the immediate and proximate areas of an active shooter situation are typically stopped because staff have to take immediate cover. Security staff should be able to answer the following questions, based on prior planning in the EOP:
- Does local law enforcement have access to life safety drawings of the facility?
- Does local law enforcement have card access for areas controlled in this fashion?
- Have the staff been trained in how to respond to these situations, including strategies like "run, hide, fight"?
- Does staff know how to deal with responding law enforcement or security personnel?

Utilizing critical incident stress debriefing during a drilled active shooter event should be considered. Some staff, based on past experiences, may need assistance in processing the drill, depending on its realism. Active shooter drills should be planned well in advance with local law enforcement.

Threat Analysis

Active Shooter Incident

When people find themselves in the vicinity of an active shooter, they must be ready to respond to the situation using one of three strategies: "run," "hide," or "fight."[1]

RUN
- Plan an escape.
- Leave personal belongings.
- Evacuate the vicinity.
- Help others leave.
- Prevent people from entering the danger zone.
- Call for help after reaching a safe location.

HIDE
- Stay out of sight.
- Block the shooter's access.
- Remain silent.

FIGHT
- As a last option, try to disable the shooter.
- React with force.
- Act quickly. This may be your only chance.

REFERENCE
1. US Department of Homeland Security. "Active Shooter: How to Respond," Accessed June 30, 2016. https://www.dhs.gov/sites/default/files/publications/active-shooter-how-to-respond-508.pdf.

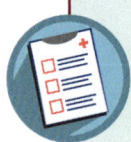

Case in Point
University of Maryland Medical Center in Baltimore Finds Itself in the Middle of a Rioting City

The Incident

The death of Freddie Gray following injuries incurred while in Baltimore police custody in April 2015 touched off more than a week of protests, civil unrest, and rioting. At the University of Maryland Medical Center, epicenter of the unrest, emergency managers were naturally concerned for the safety of patients, staff, and visitors while maintaining continuity of operations (COOP) during the challenging time.

The Response

University of Maryland Medical Center has a robust emergency management framework that stresses situational awareness and adept handling of challenges. Because incident response team members are already well versed on supporting each other for daily operations, emergency managers there began discussions about the possibility of civil unrest and the hospital's response to it days before actual conflict began. The decision was taken to initiate emergency operations early in the development of the situation.

University of Maryland Medical Center is a large academic medical center with a high-level trauma center. It is common for the R Adams Cowley Shock Trauma Center to treat victims of interpersonal violence, even at times victims from both sides of an argument, accompanied by friends and relatives with heightened emotions. So while the situations they addressed in the facility was "business as usual," the challenge of getting both patients and personnel safely to and from the hospital was unusual.

Other than a manageable patient surge and the provision of additional security measures to help safeguard those inside the facility, emergency managers identified communications, particularly rumor control and maintaining accurate situational awareness of the actual situation in the streets, as a major challenge facing the team. With angry protestors moving throughout the city, sometimes within a literal "stone's throw" of the doors of the hospital, it was critical to disseminate accurate information about developments to staff as quickly as possible to reduce anxiety and help staff stay focused.

The incident command leadership initiated an internal communications strategy that utilized an array of communications channels to keep staff and visitors apprised of developments both outside and inside the facility. These media included the hospital's intranet, e-mail blasts, messages displayed on video screens in corridors, and pager messages sent to charge nurses, who might not have access to mobile devices or other sources of e-mail. In addition, staff were gathered in regular face-to-face meetings where they were encouraged to share information, experiences, and reactions with peers and managers. This helped staff to feel supported, brought them together as teams, and facilitated communication up and down the chain of command.

> **Assessment**
> In the wake of the disturbance, the emergency management team debriefed its response to the unrest using a variety of tools, including after-action reports and online surveys. The overall assessment of the response was very good. The emergency management team recognized that prior to this incident, civil unrest had not ranked very high on their list of probable hazards, and they have since factored in an increased potential for such incidents for the future.
>
> One of the most difficult areas for the team was to decide on a balance between security and other priorities. Additional consideration will be given to questions such as, When should a security lockdown, which can adversely affect the ability to deliver care through restrictions on access and movement, be initiated? When does the need to protect staff and patients by locking doors outweigh fire safety issues? Consultation with other hospital security teams in cities facing similar challenges—be it crowds during civil unrest, political conventions, VIP visits—can provide insights going forward.

Inside Threats

Unfortunately, health care organizations are not exempt from safety threats that originate from within. Emergency management planners must include in their EOP response plans to face possible insider threats, such as staff members who may, for whatever reasons, wish to jeopardize the safety and security of their places of employment, even at the cost of their own lives. Emergency management planners, in concert with human resources managers and security staff, must consider unthinkable acts of violence as they plan responses they hope never to employ. Staff must be trained for these eventualities and be able to recognize behaviors and read indicators that may point to threats such as these. (*See* "Threat Analysis" on page 74 for situations that may lead to staff threats.)

In some cases, disgruntled staff may only wish to create confusion and chaos with no intended adverse outcomes. As part of the security threat assessment, critical areas such as the data center and communications closets may require additional security measures and redundancy to ensure COOP.

Coordinating with Law Enforcement Agencies

Organizations must, as a part of emergency planning, work with local security agencies, such as city and county police, and—through the local emergency operations center—with state and federal authorities such as the Federal Bureau of Investigation (FBI). Emergency planners need to discuss security concerns with local security agencies to identify vulnerabilities and possible mitigation activities, but it is also critical to ascertain what level of assistance the organization can expect from local law enforcement or other agencies during a disaster or terrorist incident. If, for instance, the community experiences a large civil disturbance, law enforcement resources may be otherwise occupied and not available to provide security for facilities not directly threatened by rioters.

Given that different kinds of emergencies will affect the level of security assistance available to different degrees, and the availability of assistance may change as an emergency evolves,

>
> ### Capacity Builder
> Questions to ask when considering safety precautions might include the following:
> - What types of hazardous materials and waste exist within the organization?
> - What are the specific locations of these hazardous materials and waste?
> - What are the normal procedures for securing these items?
> - What are the normal procedures for disposing of these items?
> - Have the certificates of disposal been matched up with the hazardous waste manifests?
> - How will those processes need to vary in the event of an emergency (either internal or external)? For example, what if waste cannot be collected on schedule by waste handlers?
> - What is the process in the event of evacuation?

it would benefit emergency planners to make security plans scalable, so that the organization can ramp up its own capabilities in the event that local security personnel are required elsewhere. Mutual aid agreements through local law enforcement may be of benefit, as these resources would be available for areas not impacted by the event, such as state police and county and municipal agencies in the next county.

For example, recent multisite terrorist attacks in France (November 2015) and Belgium (March 2016) are grim reminders to organizations that they must be able to stand on their own and be equipped to handle their part in escalating circumstances. An attack in one location does not rule out an attack in another location, and organizations must have plans in place and must coordinate their efforts through constant communication with community and even federal agencies. Leaders must remain on high alert for news regarding the safety and security of affected areas and any possible threat to their own organizations. This level of awareness will enable them to anticipate situations such as patient surge, as first responders to the scenes transport victims of such attacks for immediate, critical care. The circumstances of the disaster and its aftermath will likely require the complete attention of law enforcement and other agencies.

It is also likely, as was the case in the Boston Marathon bombing, that one or more of the perpetrators may be brought to the hospital for care. In such cases, additional security measures on the unit providing care to the patient are enforced by federal authorities in cooperation with local law enforcement. Access to the patient's hallway is limited for protection of staff but also for protection of the patient, as potential retaliatory threats from the community and even staff members are not uncommon in mass-casualty events. Emergency managers should also consider the discharge process for both the perpetrators and victims of violence to ensure their privacy and minimize media exposure.

It is also useful for emergency planners to learn about the ways in which local law enforcement agencies manage their own emergency response to include active shooter situations. They can meet with the chief of police, sheriff, or highway patrol leaders annually to discuss any specific concerns. They can do this by participating in local law enforcement meetings, dinners, and events and inviting their staff to participate in cooperative drills. For example, infant or pediatric abduction drills can include local law enforcement to critique and have

> ## Vulnerable Populations
>
>
>
> ### Difficulties Associated with Forensic Patients
>
> Whether during an emergency or not, some health care organizations will be called upon to deliver care to patients in law enforcement custody. Be they prison inmates whose care cannot be delivered within the facility where they are housed or suspects in need of first aid, they present an increased risk to the safety and security of staff and others in the facility. However, they are also vulnerable patients. In many cases they will be handcuffed or shackled, and they may be at risk of neglect or abuse on the basis of their situation. They may be at elevated risk for violent behavior or self-harm.
>
> Clear procedures for the handling of forensic patients are essential for minimizing danger and liability. Though forensic patients will remain in the custody of the law enforcement personnel who bring them in, security and clinical staff can take precautions to minimize risks to everyone. Security should have special procedures and a designated room set aside for the treatment of such patients. The procedures and space will help to minimize the risk of elopement and provide a safe space for searching for dangerous items like sharps, narcotics, or hazardous substances. Increased rounding may help reduce the opportunities for abuse. Staff training in de-escalation and the ability to minimize environmental stimulation can also help keep the patient calm and reduce problems. Finally, it is essential to work with local law enforcement to ensure, to the degree possible, that sufficient advance warning is given before forensic patients are brought in, and to ensure that both sides are well versed in each other's policies and procedures. The Florida Hospital Association created an online training module for accredited hospitals to orient law enforcement officers accompanying prisoners or in-custody arrestees.[1]
>
> #### REFERENCE
>
> 1. Florida Hospital Association; Florida Society for Healthcare Security, Safety, and Emergency Management Professionals. Patient Care and Prisoners. Accessed Jun 22, 2016. http://www.fha.org/showDocument.aspx?f=EMP-FT-patientcareprisoners-1152013.pps.

a female police officer act as the abductor. Bomb threat drills can also be supported by local law enforcement. Another scenario might include coordinating with agencies to expedite the transportation of staff and/or their families to the hospital when roads have been damaged or blocked or if local police or other law enforcement have set up security road blocks.

Managing Hazardous Materials and Waste

During emergency planning, organizations must identify processes for managing hazardous materials and waste during a disaster. Policies and procedures may be guided by state or local law or regulation concerning wastewater disposal or other considerations. This requirement builds on existing environment of care standards related to managing routine hazardous materials and waste risks, recognizing that the special handling required of these materials and the need to minimize the risk of unsafe use and improper disposal are particularly important to consider during emergency conditions. Some of the challenge will stem from increased volume and the need to comply with normal restrictions for disposal of hazardous materials, but some kinds of emergencies will pose novel challenges. Depending on the emergency, there may be an excess of a variety of materials, such as pharmacy waste, radioactive materials, and medical wastes such as sharps, gases, and so forth. Decontamination plans need to address the collection and disposal of water and other waste materials. Federal agencies such as the Environmental Protection Agency (EPA)[1]

Threat Analysis

Decontamination Facilities

There are several considerations related to the issue of where decontamination should take place. A decontamination facility may be internal to the facility as long as it has a direct entrance from the outside, a secondary exit to minimize cross contamination, a means to contain wastewater, and a separate ventilation system that exhausts directly to the exterior of the building. Alternatively, a number of portable outdoor decontamination units can also be effective, even in colder climates. There are pros and cons to both that the organization will have to weigh against organizational needs and the environmental threats in their community.

OUTDOOR DECONTAMINATION FACILITIES

Outdoor facilities have the advantage of keeping the contaminant totally outside the health care facility. Factors to weigh when considering the use of outdoor facilities include the following:

- Portable units: What is the cost? How much time is required and how easy is it to set up the units? Have staff been adequately drilled to ensure a quick, safe setup?

- Units connected to the facility: Is there a sheltered area or protected space (perhaps near the emergency department [ED]) where showerheads can be installed to run off of the existing plumbing? The water used for decontamination needs to be tempered so that it is not too cold or too hot for the patients. Cold water can cause hypothermia while hot water will open blood vessels, allowing for chemical absorption.

- Climate: In colder climates, can an outdoor facility be strategically located in an area adjacent to the building and connected to hot and cold running water sources? Can the exit be designed in close proximity to the entrance of the building and with a staff member waiting there with blankets? How will you heat the decontamination space? Is lighting an issue?

- Supplies and equipment: Where will required supplies and equipment be readily accessible? Are supplies and equipment stored in cleanable containers for decontamination after the incident?

- Privacy: How can privacy be protected during the decontamination process? Can otherwise uninjured victims essentially decontaminate themselves privately with a soap-and-water shower? How can you ensure a private place to disrobe and deposit contaminated clothing? How will males and females be separated? What about children? Can anyone from a distance observe the decontamination process? Are privacy barriers and/or security necessary?

- Hazardous waste disposal: How will water used for decontamination be collected and analyzed for hazardous materials prior to disposal? If portable units are used for multiple victims, how will potential wastewater overflow from the unit's base be managed? Can systems plumbed directly from the building use a drain connected to a holding tank?

INDOOR DECONTAMINATION FACILITIES

Indoor decontamination facilities overcome any climate concerns and have easy access to plumbing, but their location poses other problems. Factors to weigh when considering the use of indoor facilities include the following:

- Work flow and patient flow: What precautions are planned to avoid contaminating the ED or the facility as a whole? How have staff been trained in those precautions? How will multiple victims be accommodated? How can traffic of contaminated individuals through the building be prohibited? Can you plan for outdoor triage that allows individuals to enter directly into the decontamination facility?

- Supplies and equipment: Where will required supplies and equipment be readily accessible? Are supplies and equipment stored in cleanable containers for decontamination after the incident? Is there additional equipment needed to maintain the indoor decontamination area at negative pressure from the ED? Is the exhaust directed outside to avoid contaminating other parts of the facility?

- Hazardous waste disposal: Are portable containers for waste disposal, such as a sealable metal drum, available for disposal of contaminated items in decontamination rooms? How will contaminated water collection and disposal be handled? Does the floor pitch away from the door and toward a drain with a tank placed below to catch the used water? Can workers draw samples of wastewater for testing to identify whether the water can be discharged to the sewer or pumped out (or otherwise collected) for appropriate disposal?

ADDITIONAL DECONTAMINATION FACILITIES ISSUES

Whether facilities are located outdoors or indoors, the nature of the contaminant and the process of decontamination will influence or determine many decisions. Additional factors to consider include the following:

- Chemical incidents: What area would be most conducive to managing chemical vapors? With chemical contaminant exposure, speed is of the essence. How quickly can decontamination for chemical exposure be done? How will removal and disposal of contaminated clothing be handled as quickly as possible?

- Adjustments for containment in the facility: Can air-handling systems be isolated to prevent the spread of contaminants throughout the building? Are there certain rooms, corridors, or entrances that might be used to isolate or quarantine staff and patients, given a significant likelihood that a portion of the facility itself will be contaminated and need to be quarantined? Where will equipment such as fire-rated plastic sheeting, duct tape, and spring-loaded poles be stored to cordon off hallways or other areas and separate contaminated areas from clean ones?

- Air respirators for PPE: If air respirators are selected as personal protective equipment (PPE) for health care workers, does the design of the decontamination area include multiple connections to a dedicated air compressor or a bank of compressed air tanks? Alternatively, as long as patient care is not compromised, can the respirators be connected to the piped medical air system?

- Clean and dirty sides: Does the decontamination area include a dirty side and a clean side? How will victims and contaminated personnel and equipment be contained on the dirty side until decontaminated? Are the triage station, treatment station, and decontamination areas able to accommodate both ambulatory and nonambulatory victims (for example, patients on gurneys)? Does the plan allow victims to perform as much of the decontamination as possible themselves to decrease cross contamination?

- Clothing: Where will victims disrobe and what will they cover themselves with after decontamination? Will victims' original clothing be packaged and decontaminated or disposed of, which will help avoid further exposures of patients and staff?

- Valuables: What is the process to log in and return valuables? Where and how will the valuables be stored? Who will clean contaminated valuables? How is the determination made on which valuables patients can keep?

>
> ### Capacity Builder
>
> **Radiological and Nuclear Response**
>
> Decontamination training may be driven in part by federal requirements, or even state nuclear and radiation safety requirements for nuclear or radiological events.
>
> Statewide agencies such as the Illinois Emergency Management Agency (IEMA) have programs in place to respond to nuclear and radiological threats. In Illinois, the Radiological Task Force (RTF) contains two sections, the Radiological Emergency Assessment Center (REAC) and the Radiological Assessment Field Team (RAFT). REAC assesses the event, makes projections as to its effects, and informs the public of protective measures they should take. RAFT measures the amount of radiation in the incident area, collects and analyzes samples from the locale, and works to contain the contamination. It also coordinates with the Red Cross to set up areas to evaluate members of the public for radioactive contamination and advises health care organizations on controlling the spread of the contamination. RTF personnel are also available to assist hospitals in establishing contamination control protocols to prevent the spread of contamination throughout the facility and assist with surveys of a potentially contaminated patient, without interfering in any medical treatment.[1] Check the US Nuclear Regulatory Commission (at https://scp.nrc.gov/asdirectory.html) or your state's emergency management agency for information about similar agencies in your area.
>
> **REFERENCE**
>
> 1. Illinois Emergency Management Agency (IEMA). Nuclear Facility Safety. 2014. Accessed Jun 22, 2016. http://www.illinois.gov/iema/NRS/Pages/NuclearFacilitySafety.aspx.

Nuclear Regulatory Commission (NRC),[2] and Occupational Safety and Health Administration (OSHA)[3] provide standards and recommendations for the safe handling and disposal of hazardous materials.

Ensuring Isolation and Decontamination

Organizations planning for safety and security during emergencies must also consider radioactive, biological, infectious, and chemical isolation and decontamination needs. Contaminated patients must be segregated or isolated, decontamination procedures to treat victims and protect other patients and staff must be quickly implemented, and protocols for the safe disposal of potentially infectious or contaminated waste strictly adhered to (*see* the "Managing Hazardous Materials and Waste" section on page 73).

Isolation

An organization should plan for isolation relative to particular hazards, whether chemical, biological, or radiological in nature. Organizations should conduct assessments, in advance, of current capabilities for airborne isolation. Organizations should evaluate whether rooms on certain units or even a nursing unit can be converted to negative pressure, while identifying the potential risk and impact to high-risk populations in surrounding units such as neonatal intensive care and oncology units. Organizations should also assess and determine in advance mechanical and ventilation systems to support isolation and separation of air intake and exhaust in as many rooms as possible, if required.

Decontamination

The decontamination process involves isolating the contamination; decontaminating and treating patients; protecting staff, other patients, visitors, the organization's vehicles, and the facility itself; and reestablishing normal service. Ideally, decontamination should take place prior to patients entering the facility—for example, at the scene of the incident. However, if first responders haven't received the necessary training in decontamination, or if appropriate equipment is unavailable at the site, this may not be possible. Other factors, such as poor weather or contaminated surroundings, may necessitate conducting decontamination inside the facility. The decontamination area should have strictly controlled access and a secondary exit, a direct entrance from the outside, a means of collecting wastewater, and a separate ventilation system that exhausts directly to the exterior of the building. Portable outside decontamination units are just as effective as fixed ones. The benefit of an outdoor unit is that it provides unlimited atmosphere and minimizes building exposure to hazardous materials and waste.

In any event, first responders need to alert the organization instantly so it can arrange for trained staff to supervise the areas through which contaminated patients will be transported. Any patients or visitors must be relocated to areas of the facility separated from the decontamination zone, and staff should report to the assignments and locations suitable to their training.

Staff should have periodic training on the OSHA First Receiver guidelines in order to identify the signs and symptoms of a potentially contaminated patient (*see* pages 88–90 in Chapter 6). Registration, security, and ED staff are on the front lines and will likely be the first to identify an issue. Staff may also need cultural sensitivity training in order to accommodate religious, personal, and societal needs.

IN SUMMARY

- Crowd control during emergencies can be a challenge. The EOP should contain procedures for limiting movement into, out of, and within the facility.
- Coordinate with local law enforcement agencies and make sure that staff know what is expected of them and what responding officers will need during a security emergency.
- Safety procedures must cover isolation of infectious or potentially infectious patients or agents, decontamination of contaminated patients, and the safe storage of and access control to all hazardous materials.

REFERENCES

1. US Environmental Protection Agency. Hazardous Waste. Accessed Jun 22, 2016. https://www.epa.gov/hw.
2. US Nuclear Regulatory Commission. Radioactive Waste. (Updated: Jul 14, 2015.) Accessed Jun 22, 2016. http://www.nrc.gov/waste.html.
3. US Department of Labor, Occupational Safety & Health Administration. Materials Handling and Storage. Accessed Jun 22, 2016. https://www.osha.gov/Publications/OSHA2236/osha2236.html.

CHAPTER 6

Preparing Staff to Respond

STANDARDS FOCUS

EM.02.01.01 The organization has an Emergency Operations Plan.

EM.02.02.07 As part of its Emergency Operations Plan, the organization prepares for how it will manage staff during an emergency.

EM.02.02.13 During disasters the organization may grant disaster privileges to volunteer licensed independent practitioners.

EM.02.02.15 During disasters, the organization may assign disaster responsibilities to volunteer practitioners who are not licensed independent practitioners, but who are required by law and regulation to have a license, certification, or registration.

AT A GLANCE

- Defining staff roles
- Training staff
- Providing for staff and staff family support
- Identifying care providers
- Instituting disaster privileging
- Equipping specialized disaster response teams

WHO IS INVOLVED?

- Organization leaders
- Emergency manager
- Department heads across all departments
- Clinical and support staff
- Medical staff leadership
- Human resources
- Staff educators

Why Is This Critical?

During an emergency it is likely that staff roles will change as staff are called upon to deal with the initial effects of the emergency, and roles may shift again as an emergency unfolds. There will be little or no time to train staff for their altered roles as an emergency evolves; therefore, the proper functioning of the organization depends on staff knowing their emergency response roles ahead of time and receiving the necessary training to be able to shift from normal to emergency operations and fulfill their emergency response roles as quickly as possible during the initial minutes and hours of the response.

The emergency planning team should note that the effects of emergencies fall on care providers as well as patients. Treating trauma victims, worrying about family, worrying about physical security or safety—all of these things can adversely affect the ability of staff members to do their jobs and to cope with the increased levels of activity and long work hours that often accompany an emergency response. Organization planning and preparedness must include plans for staff support (information on the availability of child care, elder care, and pet care; access to grief counseling or pastoral care following response to a mass-casualty event; and so forth. Additional measures should be taken to ensure continuity of operations, including backup compensation plans, should computer system disruption affect payroll, downtime and recovery procedures, and redundant communications.

Key Planning Concepts for Staff Response

Making sure that the organization has sufficient numbers of staff and adequate staffing to fulfill all necessary emergency response functions is a challenge. Each staff member should be oriented to the organization's emergency operations plan (EOP), and all departments should participate in planned drills and exercises consistent with their roles in the organization's response plans. Staff with specific roles in emergency response should receive the specialized training necessary to carry out new responsibilities; training in how to fulfill these roles should be updated and refreshed regularly to retain readiness. The organization is not required to use external clinical volunteers, but if it chooses to do so, it must properly credential any clinical staff, using its regular credentialing process or the expedited process described later in this chapter.

Staff Roles

It is important to ensure that all staff members—including day-to-day support staff across all departments and the medical staff—understand their roles in an emergency. Staff must be able and ready to adjust to changes in patient volume or acuity, work procedures or conditions, and response partners within and outside the organization. Organizations should document staff roles and responsibilities in the EOP and can use a variety of formats—job action sheets, checklists, flowcharts, and so forth—for this purpose. Consider the strategies that follow to ensure that staff roles are properly documented, assigned, and understood.

Define Staff Roles and Responsibilities

Organizations will consider how staff relate to the organizational capabilities and responses before, during, and after an emergency in the six critical areas of emergency response. This amounts to an inventory of staff capabilities or an analysis of critical organizational needs and capabilities with regard to staffing. Whenever possible, the organization will assign staff to tasks that mirror what they ordinarily do at the organization. In an emergency people work best when they are performing familiar tasks or tasks for which they have been specifically trained. The EOP will provide processes for identifying and assigning staff to cover essential staff functions. It will also identify for staff the individual(s) they will need to report to in the incident command structure (ICS).

Provide Training for Staff

Provide staff with structured and recurring training on the EOP so that they can develop the following proficiencies:
- Familiarity with the overall response plan
- Knowledge of their roles in the response plan
- Knowledge of any alterations in care provision or procedures relative to patient type, equipment, supplies, communication methods, location of care, internal response team, and any external response partners
- Ability to respond rapidly at the start of an emergency and adjust individually and with their teams as the emergency evolves

The emergency manager works with staff educators, clinical staff leaders, department managers and supervisors, and local authorities and other external partners to design and provide staff education, including initial training and periodic refresher courses on areas relevant to particular types of emergencies. Such training could involve hazard identification, triage, decontamination, infection control/isolation, treatment, media and crowd control, and other appropriate topics. Developing and delivering staff education in conjunction with a health care coalition is an excellent way to provide knowledge and skills for staff that may not be routinely available in-house.

Create Quick Reference Safety Manuals

Important emergency management information should be readily available to key staff throughout the organization in both hard copy and electronic formats. Having safety reference material on hand will help to refresh regular staff on emergency roles and responsibilities. It will also provide some essential resources for staff who may work in other areas of the organization during normal operations or even volunteers who step up to fill the gaps in staff that may occur as a result of certain types of emergency situations, supporting just-in-time training.

Identify and Assign Staff Members to Cover All Essential Staff Functions under Emergency Conditions

Leadership will determine in advance the availability of staff members on short notice, how quickly they can come to the organization, and how willing they are to work overtime. Leaders should develop a protocol for alerting off-duty employees to come back to work and for providing child or elder care for them, if necessary.

To ensure continuity of operations during an event, the organization should maintain at all times a complete and current list of staff and full contact information. This information should be periodically verified so that during an emergency staff can be contacted quickly with information and instructions. When an emergency occurs, some organizations reach out to staff through automated alerts or portals and receive electronic responses confirming ability to report. In other organizations, a designated individual in each department is assigned to make calls to see which staff members can report to work and, depending on the weather and the time of year, how long it will take them to get there. If telephones are not working, the organization must use its communications backup systems to contact staff.

If staff members are unable to get to the facility for any reason, then the organization should consider its transportation options for picking them up. Having relationships with vendors may assist in this area. In some instances, staff members may not report to work because of fears of infectious disease or other related concerns about personal safety. Organizations can mitigate such concerns with proactive staff education regarding particular disease characteristics and steps the organization has taken to keep staff safe. The EOP may also outline plans to call up additional staff, such as staff from other organizations and, in extreme situations, volunteers.

Plan for the Physical Needs of Staff

The EOP will need to include provisions for respite areas, housing, food, transportation, personal hygiene, and crisis counseling for the staff. It will also consider the needs of staff families. Emergency management planning requires an awareness of logistical issues that may impact staff availability—who has school-age children or dependent elders at home, who relies on public transportation, and so forth. Planning in advance for staff support needs can help mitigate the risk of staff not reporting to or failing to remain at the organization for extended coverage during an emergency. Such needs may include planning for on-site sheltering of family members and even pets during an actual disaster.

Case in Point
Effective Disaster Response Relies on First-Class EC Training for Staff

Mark Kaldahl, currently the facility support director at Carilion Franklin Memorial Hospital in Rocky Mount, Virginia, has developed comprehensive staff training programs and materials at several institutions. He says, "Because the EC [environment of care] plays such a big role when it comes to our hospital survey, we feel that getting the information out from the very beginning, when an employee starts, is a great way to get employees introduced to it, especially in the areas of fire safety and emergency preparedness. From the very get-go in employee orientation, we talk about disaster codes and ask questions like these: What is their specific role during a fire? What is their evacuation route? Where are their assembly areas?"

Kaldahl also uses a variety of drills, booklets, and other resources to ensure that staff know their roles in an emergency and that they stay up to date with any changes. Continuous assessment of staff performance during these drills provides performance feedback to staff, but it also allows Kaldahl and others to refine training materials and methods. Things are constantly changing in the hospital environment, and this is particularly true during emergencies. An iterative approach and a commitment to constant improvement are essential.

Staff Orientation

Kaldahl's approach involves a 90-minute EC orientation session. This is an interactive presentation, using an EC information booklet and PowerPoint presentation that includes a quiz at the end to assess how well the new hires have assimilated the information. The quiz is divided into sections, each covering one of the seven areas of the EC. The results are tracked on a spreadsheet, which allows Kaldahl to assess the new hires' performance. It also allows him to see what in the presentation is working and what may need to be improved. If significant numbers of quiz takers are doing poorly on one section of the quiz, it may be the presentation or the quiz itself that needs improvement.

Kaldahl has also developed a series of department-specific EC booklets. Department leaders can use these booklets to train new staff in department-specific EC issues and challenges. Thus each new employee is taught what is expected of him or her in an emergency and what his or her department-specific responsibilities are.

Drills and Exercises

Another major component of Kaldahl's approach is frequent drilling in a variety of formats and scenarios. Drills are conducted to allow staff to put what they have learned in orientation and ongoing education to use. Though there may be organizational resistance to the increased time and expense of instituting a robust drilling program, the ongoing assessment and improvement of emergency preparedness and response pays off, as does the development of a participatory culture of safety and security.

> Kaldahl recommends conducting a variety of drills on all shifts to allow all staff to participate. This approach helps ensure that all staff are engaged in the training process and better prepares them for an emergency should one occur on their shift. Conducting drills on all shifts eliminates the problem of scheduling and paying staff overtime to attend training sessions normally conducted only during those traditional "day shift" hours. Kaldahl conducts tabletop exercises using scenarios involving threats identified in the hospital's hazard vulnerability analysis.
>
> During these exercises department leaders open up the emergency command center and work their way through the problem following the Hospital Incident Command System (HICS) format. Like the orientation process, drilling is a constantly evolving endeavor. Kaldahl is constantly assessing not only the performance of staff but the quality of the training materials and methods. For instance, while team-based exercises and training sessions work in many situations, some smaller teams may not have sufficient time to conduct them. In these cases, Kaldahl will sometimes attend department meetings and work with staff on a one-to-one basis.
>
> EC and emergency management education are essential to the continued functioning of hospitals when disaster strikes. In times of tight budgets and shrinking reimbursements, it is easy to cut back on training and drilling in favor of other priorities, but a robust staff training program is an invaluable part of emergency preparedness.

Support Staff Members in Managing Stress

Information about coping with stress should be distributed to all staff members, including how to recognize symptoms of severe stress in themselves and others and how to provide, facilitate, or request psychological support for coworkers. Plan in advance with behavioral health staff or coalition partners some strategies for providing rest breaks and psychological support for leaders and staff through long response and recovery events.

Consider how to provide access to individual or small-group counseling for staff through providers of emergency mental health services, pastoral care, or hospice grief counseling. These services will be in high demand during emergencies, particularly those involving large numbers of casualties, for patients, for their families, and for staff providing care in extreme conditions. Organizations can enhance their preparedness and their ability to care for their staff by working with mental health experts, counseling services, religious and clergy organizations, and hospice providers to plan for how these support services can be scaled up during and after emergencies.

Identify Critical Areas of Response

Depending on the type and severity of the emergency, the role of any individual staff member may be to continue to do his or her job as normal, or to perform specific emergency-related activities, on site or off site. On the other hand, specialists may be required—such as trauma and burn specialists or infection control specialists—so they, too, should be oriented in advance to their roles and responsibilities in specific emergency circumstances.

Capacity Builder

Ensuring Adequate Staffing Levels

It can be difficult to ensure adequate staffing levels at the best of times. An emergency that affects the surrounding community can present challenges that make ensuring staffing levels that much harder. Emergency planners and managers should think creatively about how to supplement their staffing levels during an emergency. The following is a list of issues to help jumpstart thinking about emergency staffing. Organizations should develop plans and protocols, testing them in drills or exercises to make sure that they can be effectively implemented during times of emergencies.

- Contacting off-duty staff to report back to work
- Educating staff on disease outbreaks and other types of emergencies
- Staff safety during emergency response and recovery, including family support
- Extending staff shifts or requesting overtime
- Canceling/postponing vacations and days off during a disaster
- Including licensed independent practitioners (generalists and specialists) in staffing plans
- Impact of state-specific laws and regulations regarding staff overtime or extended shifts
- Contingency plan for staffing if personnel are either unable or unwilling to report to work

Sample staffing strategies to assist the organization during an event may include but are not limited to the following:

- 12 hours on, 12 hours off
- Re-allocate existing staff
- Labor pool
- Overtime
- Contract staff
- Leadership backfill
- Memoranda of understanding or other agreements
- Volunteers
- Retired practitioners
- Retired staff
- Close/restrict nonessential functions
- Suspend vacations and paid time off
- Use staff from other partner facilities
- Extend shift change
- Cancel educational events/ conferences

Establish Command Structure

Essential staff members are assigned defined disaster response roles within the organization's ICS. (*See* Figure 2-5 in Chapter 2 for a sample description of staff roles and responsibilities.) Activating the ICS will eliminate confusion as to who has authority in decision making and operations. It will also show how staff are to be integrated into the broader community ICS, should that become necessary. Practicing predetermined responsibilities in training simulations will give staff opportunities to learn from any mistakes or

Threat Analysis

Debriefing to Reduce Stress

Disaster and response workers face unique stressors, which is why it is so important for health care organizations to educate staff on how to manage the stress that will naturally arise in an emergency situation. Strategies that staff members can use to manage stress during an emergency include the following:

- Developing a "buddy" system so that staff members can monitor one another's stress levels
- Encouraging and supporting their coworkers
- Limiting shifts to no more than 12 hours per day
- Taking a break when they feel that their stamina, coordination, or tolerance for irritation is diminishing
- Defusing briefly when they experience troubling incidents and after each work shift
- Making work rotations from high-stress to lower-stress functions and from the scene to routine assignments, as possible
- Talking about their emotions to process what they have seen and done
- Using available counseling assistance programs
- Participating in memorials, rituals, and use of symbols as a means to express feelings
- Taking care of themselves by eating small quantities of food and drinking water frequently
- Staying in touch with family and friends

Organizations should consider conducting separate stress debriefing sessions for leadership and general staff.

---

misunderstandings—without the stresses and uncertainties of an actual crisis situation. This practice will also make staff aware of who should report to them and to whom they should report. The ICS is instituted to keep processes running smoothly and to identify for staff the authorities and decision makers among them.

Integrate Licensed Independent Practitioners

Likewise, the EOP should spell out for licensed independent practitioners their expected roles in emergency response. These expectations are best established during regular operations when licensed independent practitioners are available to collaborate in developing patient care response plans with other clinical disciplines and departments. It can be challenging to integrate licensed independent practitioners into emergency training activities, as licensed independent practitioners may not be available for regular exercises or education sessions, and it is difficult to replicate for them the realistic constraints of resource scarcity, facility damage, or a relative lack of diagnostic or nursing support that can attend a disaster. The organization must provide opportunities for licensed independent practitioners to receive critical information and team-based practice in their response roles whenever possible, particularly considering that team composition, equipment, supplies, and space may be different from the usual care delivery setting.

Capacity Builder

Leadership Strategies

Leaders can use the following strategies, provided by Mental Health America (formerly the National Mental Health Association), after a disaster to help their workforce cope and continue to work effectively:

- Speak to the entire organization as soon as possible to express shared grief, promote available counseling services and other resources, and encourage employees to take care of themselves and their families.
- Educate supervisors and managers to recognize the signs of emotional distress and to know about available treatment resources; encourage them to seek support for themselves, or encourage staff to get treatment when necessary.
- Provide educational resources for mental health treatment.
- Facilitate communication among employees to talk and work through difficulties together.
- Consider bringing professional help on site for group meetings or individual counseling.
- Revamp your leave policy temporarily to allow time off beyond the norm for donating blood, community activity, and personal needs.
- Hold a memorial service to honor the losses of employees' loved ones or for all the victims.
- Organize community action such as a blood drive, voluntary collection fund for relief efforts, or similar activities to demonstrate the organization's commitment to helping those both within and outside the organization.
- Let business resume while acknowledging that things have changed.
- Plan for future emergencies; review the Emergency Operations Plan to address any problems that arose with the recent disaster and make sure to involve all segments of the staff in planning improvements.

Source: Adapted from National Mental Health Association. Coping with Disaster: Helping Your Workforce Cope and Return to Work. Accessed Jun 23, 2016. http://www.ncdsv.org/images/NMHA-helpingyourworkforcecopereturntowork_.pdf.

Train Volunteers

Finally, organizations should determine whether and, if so, how they will use volunteer staff—clinical or nonclinical—in emergency response. Sources of emergency volunteers can be the organization's usual volunteers, volunteers from the organization's parent company or sister companies, additional volunteers from the community (for example, ham radio operators), nonclinical and clinical peers from the health care coalition, registered volunteers from regional, state, or federal disaster response teams (for example, a Disaster Medical Assistance Team [DMAT]).

Potential volunteers should be contacted in advance where possible and train and exercise for their roles in an emergency response with the organization. Organizations will need to create or obtain ahead of time quick reference tools that can be used to provide just-in-time training on emergency response tasks and reporting structures to help coordinate volunteers during the emergency, including spontaneous volunteers such as medical staff displaced from another facility who could be integrated into the emergency response. (The expedited credentialing of volunteers who are licensed independent practitioners, and licensed clinical volunteers who are not licensed independent practitioners, is described beginning on page 94 in this chapter.)

Staff Training

Staff orientation and training are essential parts of the emergency planning process, not only required by Joint Commission standards, but as a way to make sure that all staff understand their responsibilities in emergency response, can respond quickly at the start of an actual emergency, and can work with effectiveness and flexibility with their coworkers as the emergency evolves. An EOP should outline who is responsible for staff education at the organization. By conducting comprehensive training with periodic refresher classes, organizations can help staff deliver the best care to disaster victims and other patients given the circumstances of the emergency. Senior leaders (operational and clinical) must support emergency management training as an organizationwide effort, and plan and budget for such training accordingly.

The EOP is developed in collaboration with all departments to ensure that it leverages all the organization's capabilities with respect to staff, supplies, and space, and reflects the patient population(s) that would require care during an emergency. Similarly, department heads and area managers should participate where possible in the design and delivery of emergency operations education. Training sessions should include the appropriate clinical, operational, and facilities subject matter experts. For example, if an organization is determined to be at high risk for earthquakes, clinical and nursing staff may need extra training in the triage and treatment for crash injuries and other kinds of trauma, and these classes should be led by staff with appropriate experience and training. Organizations must decide which sessions will be conducted on a quarterly, biannual, and annual basis. To keep the lessons fresh and in the forefront of everyone's minds, some organizations divide training topics into 12 modules that are presented on a monthly basis and may include disaster drill scenarios based on these needs.

Formats for training vary almost as much as the individual roles and responsibilities during an emergency. Classroom or seminar settings can range from two-hour lectures to workshops that can last for several days. Or training can be provided via satellite broadcasts, webinars, podcasts, "town hall" meetings, or live lectures. Many organizations employ a "train-the-trainer" model that involves training a small group of employees who then train coworkers. Another format option is a self-study program, either computer or manual based, that staff can complete at home or in another setting.

In-house instructors are not the only option for leading staff training sessions. Other individuals who might be involved include representatives of the local Office of Emergency Management, regional ASPR (Assistant Secretary for Preparedness and Response) groups, state Occupational Safety and Health Administration (OSHA) office, local police or fire departments, emergency medical services or public health representatives, or equipment and pharmaceutical manufacturers.

Training for Specific Situations

All staff members should receive education in the skills required to perform their roles in an emergency. Depending on their role, the education may include risk identification, triage, decontamination, infection control and isolation, treatment, shelter in place, and evacuation.

Risk Identification

Staff training should include how staff are to identify certain key risks or how to call certain suspected risks to the attention of their supervisor or designated staff. The type of training will depend on the staff member's role and responsibilities during an emergency. Some risks are weather related; designated staff monitoring external authorized news sources can effectively identify such risks, including sometimes their timing and impact. All personnel should know how to recognize an active shooter situation and how to react, including survival strategies such as "run, hide, fight." Other risks, such as the risk of infectious disease, require general precautions that all staff should take with all patients, and special procedures around patients suspected of having or being at risk of having an infectious disease.

In these cases, and in cases such as suspected environmental exposure to dangerous chemicals, radiological substances, or other toxins, specialized staff must screen and assess patients based on risk. As per the requirements of OSHA, the Centers for Disease Control and Prevention (CDC), and other authorities, the EOP should include policies that provide safety protections for staff. These policies should guide staff training, including the provision of equipment and practice in facilities with specialized stipulations. These components of training enable staff to face situations such as the identification, decontamination, and isolation of patients at risk.

Triage

Regular triage rules for providing the standard of care to each individual still apply, even when the emergency temporarily alters the availability of usual staff, supplies, or space, or an influx of patients results in a delay of care or prioritizing patients based on acuity. The triage plan in the EOP describes how, where, and by whom all arriving patients will be assessed and treated, discharged, or transferred. Staff should know how to respond quickly and effectively to help a large influx of patients at one time. (Crisis standards of care, which are applied only in rare circumstances, are described in the "Special Report" section in Chapter 2)

Decontamination

The EOP should address decontamination during emergencies, including who carries it out and where on the organization grounds it is performed (described more fully in the "Threat Analysis" section in Chapter 5). Attention to space, equipment, communication, and patient flow are essential for a safe and effective decontamination process.

OSHA's Hazardous Waste Operations and Emergency Response (HAZWOPER) standard requires health care organizations to train workers to perform their anticipated job duties—including decontamination—without endangering themselves or others. The extent and content of the training will depend on the employee's designated role under the EOP.

Employees designated as "first receivers" (that is, those whose duties would bring them into direct contact with patients presenting prior to decontamination—for example,

Vulnerable Populations

Organizations will want to consider staff training related to specific populations served by the organization. For example, a Medicare/Medicaid-based nursing care center providing services to residents with Alzheimer's disease or a hospital with a large pediatric unit will want to train the leaders responsible for implementing the Emergency Operations Plan in how to effectively train staff to evacuate such individuals. Transporting confused elderly residents or frightened children requires sensitivity to the issues involved with their specific care needs and the special vulnerabilities of those patients. The effectiveness of educational efforts might be addressed through ongoing monitoring of staff knowledge and skills and level of staff participation.

Other vulnerable populations whose needs should be taken into account in emergency planning—depending on the type of organization or facility—include patients with mental illness or dementia, those who do not speak English or have limited English proficiency, oxygen-dependent patients and those with chronic illnesses such as kidney or heart disease, and those at higher risk due to health disparities related to poverty, race, immigration status, or other factors. Many of these individuals rely on community health entities such as community health centers, kidney dialysis centers, faith communities, and social service organizations for care and services. Emergency managers may want to consider reaching out to leaders in such organizations throughout the community during the planning process. Relationships with these entities can both help emergency planners understand the special needs of the groups they serve and serve as the basis for community health care coalitions through which an organization can solicit specialized expertise during emergencies.

decontamination rapid-response staff, clinicians who triage and/or stabilize victims before and after decontamination, security staff who would work within the decontamination zone) must have OSHA first responder operations level training. The content of this training may be modified to exclude topics and competencies not germane to the health care setting, and instead focus on competencies such as decontamination procedures, use of personal protective equipment (PPE), and recognition of signs and symptoms of exposure to an array of hazardous materials. Any staff member with a designated role within the decontamination zone should receive this training. In smaller organizations this may include staff from departments across the organization whose emergency response roles include setting up and operating decontamination equipment or facilities.

Other employees who might come into contact with patients presenting at the emergency department (ED) or other areas of the health care organization (for example, ED staff, security, patient intake and tracking clerks, front desk clerks) must also receive OSHA first responder awareness level training. This training focuses more on identifying possible exposure patients and notifying the appropriate parties so that patients can be quickly isolated and decontaminated.

The more comprehensive HAZWOPER technician level training may be required if there is significant risk of a hazardous materials spill or leak on the organization premises. Other staff and those whose presence or involvement cannot be anticipated ahead of time may receive just-in-time training on the necessary skills, such as use of PPE, as needed.

Annual refresher training is required by OSHA as well. In addition, bear in mind that these are the basic minimum standards. More extensive training may be required under state law or regulation, and, in some states, ASPR grants may require certain numbers of staff with specific training levels.

Infection Control/Isolation

The organization must educate staff about the appropriate infection control precautions they should take when treating individuals with suspected or confirmed communicable diseases, including bioterrorism-related illnesses or a novel emerging infectious disease. For staff with certain functions, this would include standard contact precautions and droplet or airborne precautions. Health care workers should also receive training in proper sanitation measures to contain the spread of infection. (For Joint Commission standards on infection control, consult the "Infection Prevention and Control" chapter of the applicable accreditation manual.) Training can be supplemented with signs, posters, pamphlets, or other materials designed to foster an ongoing awareness of infection control procedures. (*See* Figure 6-1 for an example.)

In addition, some organizations collaborate with local departments of health and others to conduct syndromic surveillance. Syndromic surveillance uses data, such as numbers of patients presenting with flulike symptoms or health care worker absenteeism rates, to help identify infectious disease outbreaks earlier.

Treatment

An emergency requires staff to provide the usual standard of care under often adverse circumstances—for an influx of patients; for a patient population not normally treated in such volume (for example, pediatric burn patients); in a damaged facility; without all the usual supplies, staff support, or space; or in escalating conditions (for example, flood then power failure). Staff members will require training individually and in teams in providing care, treatment, and service safely in less than optimal conditions. Staff may require training in treating illnesses and injuries they might not see on a regular basis or might have never seen. As a result of a bioterrorism attack, for example, an infectious disease that was almost eradicated or is very rare, such as smallpox or the plague, could resurface. Staff could be treating mass casualties or triaging an influx of infectious patients. In addition to treating the actual victims of an emergency, staff should understand how to provide this treatment without compromising the care of others in the organization.

Although The Joint Commission does not mandate the frequency of training in any of the competencies related to emergency response, certain competencies may be governed by regulatory agencies, and certifications may be required, which may require periodic retraining. For instance, OSHA requires annual retraining in decontamination protocols for certain kinds of responders, as described previously.

Shelter in Place

Many disasters will require staff and patients to shelter in place. Staff will need training and drilling in the procedures for securing themselves, patients, critical supplies, and so on during such events. Examples include a violent storm striking the area and creating conditions that are not safe for discharging patients or allowing staff to leave at the end of their shifts; the facility being placed on lockdown during an active shooter situation; and a train derailment

Figure 6-1. Evaluation and Management of Patients

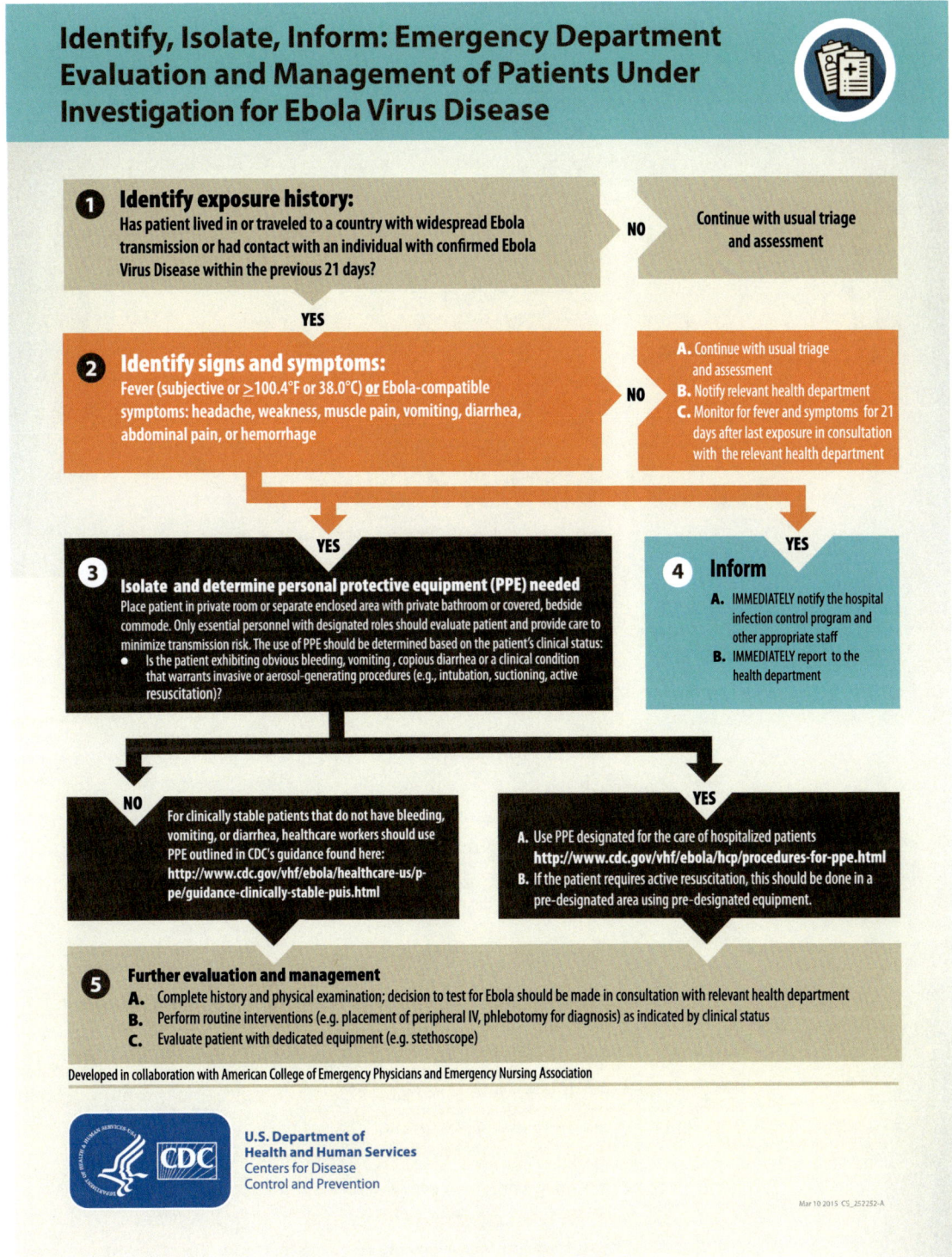

Figure 6-1 provides a model to identify signs and symptoms of patients with infectious diseases.

Source: Centers for Disease Control and Prevention. Identify, Isolate, Inform: Emergency Department Evaluation and Management of Patients Under Investigation for Ebola Virus Disease. Mar 10, 2015. Accessed Jun 23, 2016. www.cdc.gov/vhf/ebola/pdf/ed-algorithm-management-patients-possible-ebola.pdf.

Case in Point
Deadly EF5 Tornado Ravages Hospital and Requires Evacuation

For days following, headlines like "Mercy Hospital Joplin in Direct Path of Deadly EF5 Tornado" and "Tornado's Wake Leaves Disaster Zone" recounted the devastation caused by the EF5 tornado—one of the most powerful ever recorded—that ravaged Joplin, Missouri, on May 22, 2011. Mercy (formerly St. John's Regional Medical Center) sat directly in the cyclone's path, testing its staff, patients, and emergency preparedness.

Because meteorologists had forecast severe storms, Mercy sounded its "Prepare for Condition Gray" code earlier in the day. Staff alerted patients and visitors about the imminent storm, closed curtains and blinds, and prepositioned chairs in hallways as they practiced in drills. When the storm approached, Mercy escalated to "Execute Condition Gray," and staff evacuated patients into hallways, closing doors behind them. With 20 minutes' warning, patients and staff took cover before the EF5 tornado ripped through the hospital.

In moments, the roof collapsed, recounts Dennis Manley, RN, HRM, CPHQ, director, Quality and Risk Management, Mercy Hospital Joplin. The severe storm blew out most windows; tore doors off hinges; caused sprinkler, sewer, and gas pipes to burst; and destroyed the main oxygen tanks. Tiles, wiring, and cables fell and hung loose from the ceiling. "The hallways were filled with debris," says Manley. Fire doors had closed automatically, and debris, including doors and equipment, had blown against them, making it difficult to move around. The tornado destroyed redundant systems and backups to backups. There were no radios, telephones, Internet, or intercom. With the exception of some limited texting and cell phone use, there was no communication in the building or with the community. "We lost all functions of the hospital," says Manley. "When you lose backups, you have to rely on training, drills, and your staff's knowledge, responses, and reactions to take care of the situation. Staff relied on knowledge and expertise to know what to do and how to evacuate patients."

Robert Dodson, MD, chief of medical staff and trauma surgeon, Mercy Hospital Joplin, who was home when the tornado hit, headed to the hospital within minutes of the storm and described the approaching scene as a disaster zone. "Curtains flew out of windows. Liquid oxygen tanks spewed vapor. Damaged cars littered the grounds and were even piled up in places," says Dodson. "Most people couldn't get close to the hospital. Some staff walked to the site."

The Mercy incident command center and its alternative location were both destroyed in the storm. "We couldn't even go to a disaster trailer. It was gone," comments Dodson. "We found it a week later across the street in Cunningham Park."

Evacuating, Triaging, and Relocating Patients

After the storm passed, staff began evacuating patients to three central collecting points outside the hospital. At each collecting point, the sheriff's department informed patients and staff about next steps. Within 90 minutes of the event, all patients and staff were out of the building. Less critical patients then went to the Brady Rehabilitation Building on Mercy's campus, which sustained some damage but had a working generator. The most critical patients were brought to neighboring Freeman Health System (Freeman). Because there were a limited number of available ambulances, patients were transported using SUVs and pickup trucks from community members and off-duty staff who arrived at the hospital to help. Nurses and paramedics accompanied patients and brought with them life-sustaining equipment, such as Ambu® bags, to provide care to patients while in transit. When the most critical patients were out of the building, staff worked on placing the less severe patients in the Brady Building. Most of these patients were transported in school buses to Memorial Hall, the alternative care site and triage center in Joplin. After all patients were moved, staff and community helpers then hauled equipment, such as crash carts and IVs, back to Memorial Hall. MRI and CT scan units were also set up at Memorial Hall.

Continuing to Provide Patient Care

Mercy's patients were displaced, and it had no building. How would it continue providing patient care? Fortunately, Mercy had implemented an electronic health record (EHR) system on May 1, 2011, just three weeks prior to the storm. Because of this EHR system, all patient records were saved. Mercy Hospital Joplin is part of Mercy Health System, headquartered in the St. Louis area, which was able to access all records online, send them to the next care providers and/or receiving hospitals, and track where each patient went, which took several days. For patients who remained in the Mercy system, records were easily accessible by computer; otherwise, records were printed and then forwarded to the receiving health care organization.

Do What You Practice

According to Manley, the staff's reaction was the most positive aspect of the emergency. Because of drilling, education, and continual training, staff knew what to do and acted appropriately. "The evacuation process was organized and efficient," says Manley. "The reaction from the staff was quite phenomenal."

Although one visitor and five patients who were in critical condition when the storm hit perished during the tornado, it is probable that lives were spared due to the efficient and competent response of Mercy's staff.[1] Because of the staff's emergency management training, according to Manley and Dodson, the hospital was evacuated in 90 minutes and no injuries were sustained by staff or patients during the evacuation. Staff also knew the location of the alternative care site, so they did not need to be told where to go. In addition to the staff's response to executing the emergency plan, equipment and supply vendors were part of the plan and responded quickly by sending new equipment and supplies as early as that evening.

REFERENCE

1. Nurse.com. Preparation Pays Off in Joplin. Domrose C. Jul 11, 2011. Accessed Jun 23, 2016. https://www.nurse.com/blog/2011/06/06/preparation-pays-off-in-joplin-5/.

that leaks a chemical plume. Staff should be familiar with shelter-in-place procedures and protocols for both disaster- and security-related scenarios as detailed in the EOP. This knowledge will enable them to protect themselves and patients and continue to deliver care. The responsibilities of caring for special populations require staff to be provided with special training. For example, one of the challenges faced by staff in long term memory support facilities when sheltering in place includes the need for staff to have special training, procedures, and environmental support in preventing wandering and in keeping patients calm.

Evacuation
Although complete evacuation of a facility does not happen often, when it occurs as a result of a catastrophe, the organization and its staff must be prepared to efficiently carry out the process. Otherwise, the evacuation adds to the emergency and can itself put patients and staff at risk. Staff members must know their specific roles and responsibilities in preparing for building evacuation, know the location of equipment for evacuating or transporting patients, and understand how to carry out the actual evacuation. Issues to be managed during an evacuation include the transportation of patients, their medications and equipment, and staff.

Identifying Care Providers
During an emergency situation, a health care organization may be dealing with a chaotic environment—damaged facilities, an influx of patients and visitors, extraordinary time pressures, and many other factors. These circumstances make it important to identify care providers and other personnel assigned to particular areas during emergencies. Organizations can meet this requirement in a variety of ways, such as by using identification cards, wristbands, vests, hats, badges, or computer printouts.

Disaster Volunteer Privileging
When there is an increased demand for care and services during emergency operations, the organization may choose to extend privileges to licensed independent practitioners and other clinical volunteers, and the exigencies of the moment may require organizations to expedite the normal privileging and credentialing process. However, the organization's leadership will still need to plan in advance for verifying their qualifications and credentials, and medical staff must plan in advance to provide proper oversight of their actions and duties.

Modified privileging may only occur after the activation of the EOP and the organization has determined that it is unable to meet patient needs. After verifying credentials, the organization's EOP will have a plan in place to assign appropriate disaster responsibilities. (*See* Figure 6-2 on page 96 for a better understanding of the processes of disaster credentialing and disaster responsibilities.) As always, the goal in any health care situation—emergency and otherwise—is to provide safe and uncompromised care to patients.

Credentialing Licensed Independent Practitioners
Before any licensed independent practitioner is allowed to function as a volunteer licensed independent practitioner, he or she must present a valid government-issued picture identification, and his or her license to practice for verification purposes. The organization can verify this license in a number of ways, though contacting the licensing authority or viewing the actual license, if possible, are preferable methods, or by reviewing proof that he or she is authorized to provide care as part of a Disaster Medical Assistance Team (DMAT), Disaster Mortuary Assistance Team (DMORT), or Medical Reserve Corps (MRC), or under other

> ## Setting Spotlight
>
>
>
> ### Ambulatory Health Care
> Ambulatory health care settings cover a wide range of services, from clinical settings, such as pediatric, geriatric, and obstetric and gynecological practices, to critical services such as those offered by cancer centers, urgent care centers, and dialysis centers. In an emergency, many, if not all of these services may rely as much on patient education as they do on educated, prepared staff.
>
> Take, as an example, a dialysis center that may no longer afford safe patient care. Perhaps utilities fail or resources such as water become scarce or contaminated. Staff may be limited and yet have a number of patients to care for simultaneously. An emergency may require immediate evacuation. Dialysis patients, however, cannot just stand up and leave the facility unassisted. How can dialysis centers prepare for circumstances such as this and plan for the protection of their patients?
>
> Ambulatory organizations can provide patient education. Whether in an ambulatory setting or in their homes, patients—like staff—should be trained on how to care for themselves. Organizations can offer patients information, such as instruction brochures, to study. They can create posters with directions and make sure that they are accessible throughout the facility. They can also upload reference materials to a website or portal. And they can walk patients through a physical drill of what they might have to do to care for themselves in a circumstance when they won't have staff assistance.
>
> In the event that patients are stranded in their homes, without transportation, or unable to receive services from a damaged or evacuated facility, they must have some basic knowledge of what to do until services are up and running again. The organization might consider furnishing patients with paperwork identifying them as dialysis patients and detailing their needs, should they require help at another location. Staff might also provide patients with contact numbers of additional sites of service. Finally, they might prepare patients to care for their own physical needs and equipment and—during normal operating circumstances—give them supplies to keep in their homes as a backup kit.

special privileging mechanisms. In any case, primary source verification of licensure must occur as soon as the disaster is under control, or within 72 hours of the licensed independent practitioner presenting him or herself at the health care organization, whichever comes first. If verification is not possible within 72 hours of the practitioner's arrival, the reasons why should be documented, along with evidence of the attempt(s) to verify, and evidence of the practitioner's demonstrated ability to continue providing care, treatment, or service.

The medical staff oversees all volunteer licensed independent practitioners, and each volunteer licensed independent practitioner's performance should be reviewed no more than 72 hours following the granting of privileges. At that point, staff leaders will determine whether or not to continue to extend those privileges.

Credentialing Licensed Clinical Volunteers Who Are Not Licensed Independent Practitioners
Licensed volunteers who are not licensed independent practitioners must go through a similar vetting process to be granted clinical responsibilities during a disaster. As with licensed independent practitioners, each nonlicensed independent practitioner volunteer must present photo identification and proof of licensure or proof that he or she is authorized

Figure 6-2. Granting Disaster Privileges and Assigning Disaster Responsibilities

Two Processes		
	Process 1: *Granting disaster privileges*	**Process 2:** *Assigning disaster responsibilities*
Standard	EM.02.02.13	EM.02.02.15
Clinician type	Licensed independent practitioners	Other practitioners who require a license, certification, or registration but do not practice independently
Examples (depending on state law)	Physicians, physician assistants, nurse practitioners, dentists, nurse midwives	Registered nurses, dietitians, social workers, laboratory technicians, medical assistants, licensed practical nurses, physical therapists
Process requirements	Granting disaster privileges as defined in the medical staff privileging process	Assigning disaster responsibilities based on hospital policies and applicable job descriptions
Responsible entities	Medical staff; person(s) designated by the medical staff	Human resources or other assigned department

Figure 6-2 illustrates the differences in granting disaster privileges and assigning disaster responsibilities.

to provide care as part of a DMAT, DMORT, or MRC, or under other special privileging mechanisms.

The organization must oversee the performance of licensed volunteers who are not licensed independent practitioners. The organization defines in writing the methods and practices of that oversight. A good way for testing the plans for using volunteers is to hold training exercises in which medical staff work with "volunteers" in simulated emergency scenarios to identify the challenges that occur through volunteer assistance. The best time to navigate these processes and identify any challenges is in training exercises, in order for involved staff to be fully prepared to make effective use of volunteers.

IN SUMMARY

- Make sure each and every staff member knows his or her responsibilities during an emergency. Train staff to perform their disaster roles and drill them often to help create a culture of safety and teamwork.

- Train staff with responsibility for special populations to handle the particular challenges in caring for those patients during an emergency and possible evacuation.

- Create a system for recruiting and managing volunteers and for special disaster credentialing to ensure adequate staffing levels during patient surges and other emergency situations that are labor intensive.

CHAPTER 7

Safeguarding Utilities

> **STANDARDS FOCUS**
>
> **EM.02.01.01** The organization has an Emergency Operations Plan.
>
> **EM.02.02.09** As part of its Emergency Operations Plan, the organization prepares for how it will manage utilities during an emergency.

AT A GLANCE
- Planning for utilities failure
- Managing utilities during an emergency

WHO IS INVOLVED?
- Administrative leaders
- Emergency manager
- Facilities manager
- Clinical engineering
- Information management
- Medical staff
- Safety officer

Why Is This Critical?

Loss of utilities—in particular, prolonged loss of electrical power—can result in the need to modify how care is delivered, to cease services, or to evacuate the facility. Electrical power enables the organization to run diagnostic equipment and patient monitors, perform certain clinical procedures, and provide light, climate control, refrigeration, and myriad other services and functions. In addition to electrical power, it will be difficult for the organization to continue providing all essential care and services if there is a prolonged disruption in the supply of water (both potable and nonpotable), fuel for building operations and vehicles, medical gas, or the operation of ventilation and vacuum systems.

Key Planning Concepts for Utilities

Utilities are essential to the proper operation of the environment of care and significantly contribute to effective, safe, and reliable care. Yet utilities are often impacted during internal or external emergencies, both natural and human-made. Managing utilities cannot be compromised, or adverse events could endanger the safety of patients.

Planning for Utilities Failure

Emergencies may stress, damage, destroy, or otherwise prevent access to utility systems. Electrical sources to the facility are vulnerable to fires, generalized outages, downed lines, and so on. Water systems can be overwhelmed and/or contaminated through industrial and natural sources, malfunctioning treatment systems, and even acts of terrorism. Stringent training in treating and identifying contamination of water is crucial. Its countless uses in the facility are critical to high-quality patient care (*see* the "Threat Analysis" section on page 100 and the "Capacity Builder" section on page 102).

Emergencies could occur internally. All of these systems are also vulnerable to intentional damage or sabotage. So managing utilities due to various emergencies is not limited to external factors.

Because utility systems are critical to the continued services provided by hospitals and other health care facilities, The Joint Commission requires organizations to develop written contingency plans for how they will manage utility services relative to the environment of care, including clinical interventions.

Emergencies present another level of risk to the physical environment, and organizations are required to identify alternative means of providing for the following services, among others:
- Electricity
- Water for consumption and essential care activities
- Water for equipment and sanitation
- Fuel for building operations, generators, and transportation
- Other systems deemed essential, such as medical gas and vacuum systems; heating, ventilating, and air-conditioning (HVAC) systems; vertical and horizontal transport systems; steam for sterilization; and so on

Each of these systems needs to be considered across all phases of emergency management.

Mitigation

The maintenance and upgrading of equipment—for example, equipment that relies on an electrical system—are essential to proper function. Equipment manufacturers may provide recommendations and preventative measures regarding the longevity and effectiveness of the equipment they deliver. However, decisions to maintain and upgrade equipment may be a coordinated effort that includes monitoring and assessment by both clinical and engineering staff. In addition, departmental staff can offer valuable input in the maintenance of equipment systems. They have daily contact with patients who rely on equipment to sustain their health. Because these staff members are frequent users of equipment systems, they provide essential information regarding the effectiveness of and problems in the regular use of the equipment.

The emergency management team may consider upgrades as an opportunity to better integrate backup sources and distribution systems—such as a generator and normal electrical infrastructure—to maintain safe and effective operations. Hardware and software for monitoring emergency power systems not only help manage power supply and demand in an emergency, they can allow remote system testing for emergency preparedness and compliance purposes. More and more, organizations budget and manage their utilities and their resources and assets with a movement toward self-sustainment and resilience in advance of an emergency and its requirements.

To address the need for nonpotable water, some organizations have both potable and nonpotable wells on site. In addition, some organizations plan for suppliers to bring tankers of water to the facility if normal sources are not available. Organizations should consider, though, what will happen if tankers cannot reach the organization due to roads blocked by debris or treacherous driving conditions caused by snow or ice.

CHAPTER 7 | Safeguarding Utilities

Figure 7-1. **Emergency Power Preparation Checklist**

An Emergency Power Preparation Checklist

In addition to the inspection, testing, and maintenance requirements for emergency power systems, The Joint Commission supports the following proactive steps to avoid adverse events caused by an emergency electrical power system failure:

☐ Perform a gap analysis on the emergency power system that compares the critical equipment and systems needed in an extended emergency against the equipment and systems actually on the emergency power system.

☐ Use disaster scenario planning to identify critical systems that could potentially be lost (for example, potable water or elevators).

☐ Maintain a complete, labeled inventory of all emergency power systems and the loads they serve.

☐ Provide competency training and testing for all operators and others responsible for system maintenance of the emergency power supply system.

☐ Test generator fuel oil, track expiration dates, and replace stale fuel oil not consumed within its storage life.

☐ Ensure that engineering staff communicate the capabilities and limitations of the emergency power supply system to the organization's management and clinical leaders. These communications should cover how long emergency power will be available, how long it will take the generators to provide power if and when the utility company's power is lost, and what locations within the facility will and will not be powered by the emergency power.

☐ Establish contingency plans for clinicians to follow during brief or sustained losses of emergency power and include this information as part of the orientation and periodic continuing educational activities for medical and other clinical staff.

☐ Have plans in place for rapid deployment of battery-powered equipment, such as portable suction units, in case of a power failure.

☐ Regularly assess critical equipment to ensure that it is plugged into backup power outlets.

☐ Create a "disaster bin" that contains flashlights, extension cords, and so on.

Source: The Joint Commission. *Sentinel Event Alert*, Issue 37: Preventing adverse events caused by emergency electrical power system failures. Accessed Nov 20, 2013. http://www.jointcommission.org/sentinel_event_alert_issue_37_preventing_adverse_events_caused_by_emergency_electrical_power_system_failures/.

Figure 7-1 provides a checklist of activities organizations can perform to ensure that their utilities systems are prepared to withstand emergencies.

Threat Analysis

Precautions During Water Contamination Emergencies

AVOIDING DANGER ZONES

Careful preparations need to be made regarding the following activities and areas during a water contamination emergency:

- **Drinking water**—During a boil water notice or a "Do not drink the water" notice, take the following actions:
  - Discontinue the consumption of tap water.
  - Turn off ice makers, soda fountains, drinking fountains, and any other equipment that requires water that might be ingested.
  - Label all remaining water sources, "Do not drink."
  - Provide bottled water, juices, or soft drinks for patients and staff.
  - Use only bagged ice from a source unaffected by the contaminated water alert.

- **Food preparation**—During a boil water advisory or a boil water notice, take the following actions:
  - Heat food prepared using tap water to at least 165°F (73.9°C) before serving.
  - Serve prepackaged foods and fruits that are normally peeled before eating.
  - Require food service workers to use hand sanitizers after washing their hands during a boil water notice or a "Do not consume" notice.
  - Discontinue food preparation activities that involve the use of tap water.
  - Serve only prepackaged foods obtained from approved commercial sources not affected by the boil water notice and fruit that is normally peeled before eating.

- **Dishwashing**—According to Occupational Safety and Health Administration (OSHA) 29 CFR 1910 General Industry Standards, nonpotable water shall not be used for washing any portion of a person, cooking or eating utensils, or clothing.[1] During a boil water advisory or a boil water notice for total coliform contamination, take the following actions:
  - Use only commercial dishwashers equipped with hot water (180°F [82.2°C]) sanitizing cycles for washing dishes.
  - In facilities not equipped with 180°F dishwashers, use only single-service eating and drinking utensils.
  - Use disposable single-service utensils and packaged foods (during a boil water notice for fecal coliform contamination or a "Do not consume" notice).

- **Hand washing**—If contaminated water is used for hand washing, a further step must be taken to inactivate bacteria that the water might leave on your hands. For health care workers, this means using alcohol-based hand sanitizer. In situations in which the hands are heavily soiled and need to be washed with soap and water before they can be sanitized, staff should do the following:
  - Wash hands with soap and water, dry thoroughly, and then sanitize using an alcohol-based hand sanitizer (if water is available) or
  - Wash hands with soap and bottled water, dry thoroughly, and then sanitize using alcohol based hand sanitizer (if water is not available)

> - **Bathing**—The OSHA recommendation to refrain from washing any portion of a person would also apply during a boil water notice or a do not drink the water notice. During contaminated water emergencies, take the following actions:
>   – Bathe patients using disposable bathing washcloths.
>   – Bathe patients with a disposal cleanser that can be used without water.
>
> **REFERENCE**
> 1. US Occupational Safety and Health Administration. 29 CFR 1910, Subpart J: General Environmental Controls. [1910.141(b)(2)(iii)]. Accessed Jun 24, 2016. https://www.osha.gov/pls/oshaweb/owadisp.show_document?p_table=STANDARDS&p_id=9790.

Preparedness

Planning for and drilling on primary and backup systems failures will help identify gaps in planning and increase the efficiency with which facilities managers are able to diagnose, mitigate, and solve problems, as well as to identify and implement alternatives. Building capacity and resource identification into the preparedness efforts is important. Some organizations plan utilities shutdowns to occur with system upgrades and mitigation activities as an opportunity to drill utilities failures and identify added measures that can be implemented early.

However an organization decides to simulate outages, it is important for the organization to understand its baseline for utilization—how much and how quickly the organization uses water, fuel, and other critical resources during normal and peak times—to better anticipate needs during the emergency. It is also important to identify alternative sources of critical utilities ahead of time and negotiate agreements or memoranda of understanding with those suppliers to provide for the organization's needs in an emergency. If the emergency electrical system fails, where will the facility acquire mobile generators? Where will the organization turn if it needs to have water, fuel, or medical gas delivered by truck? Organizations need to consider these and similar questions and contact suppliers within their systems and coalitions and within their communities, as well as outside their local area, in case a communitywide disaster prevents local suppliers from meeting demand. For example, most codes require only limited elevators to be on backup power; organizations may need to develop contingencies to make sure that backup power may be available to power all elevators to support patient evacuation, delivery of water to floors, and other scenarios.

Managing Utilities During an Emergency

Organizations should develop systems for monitoring critical utilities and the functioning of primary and backup systems for them. Effective emergency response requires emergency managers, building engineers, and other staff to anticipate and monitor utility disruptions so they can support senior leadership in making informed decisions relative to patient care and environmental safety. Key staff must be aware of the physical location of affected utilities in the facility so they can get there as quickly as possible to begin response procedures.

The Emergency Operations Plan (EOP) should also contain explicit instructions for how information about electrical and water systems will be communicated up the incident command structure and for how the organization will source fuel, water, and other supplies and monitor their use throughout response and recovery. Consider plans with vendors for delivering a temporary system to deliver essential services, such as a backup generator, and

Capacity Builder

Managing Risks Associated with an Interrupted or Contaminated Water Supply

Interruption or contamination of a water supply can be caused by a range of incidents, including natural disasters, malfunctioning wastewater treatment systems, sewer overflows, manufacturing processes, and acts of terrorism.

When water interruption disasters occur, health care organizations must be prepared to handle the emergency with minimal disruption to normal patient care activities. According to the Centers for Disease Control and Prevention, water may not be available for the following vital activities[1]:

- Hand washing and hygiene
- Drinking at faucets and fountains
- Food preparation
- Flushing toilets and bathing patients
- Laundry
- Sterilization of surgical instruments
- Reprocessing of medical equipment
- Patient care
- Fire suppression sprinkler systems
- Water-cooled medical gas and suction compressors
- Heating, ventilating, and air-conditioning
- Decontamination/hazmat response

Consequently, the organization must have a plan in place to protect occupants from the harmful effects of contaminated water.

Water Contaminants

When the water source becomes contaminated, the health care organization is advised not to use the water unless it is first boiled or disinfected before use. This notification will often be made either by the facility's water supplier or the local health department. The reason these warnings are issued can usually be summed up in one portentous word: coliforms. Coliforms are bacteria that are present in the digestive tracts of humans and animals and are found in their wastes. They are also found in plant and soil material.

Other water contaminates include the following[2]:

- Organic compounds, such as pesticides, herbicides, insecticides, and fungicides
- Volatile organic chemicals (VOCs)
- Inorganic compounds such as arsenic, barium, chromium, lead, mercury, and silver
- Radioactive elements such as radon or alpha/beta emitters

Advisories, Notifications, and Warnings

Government agencies issue advisories, notifications, and warnings, which are typically broadcast by the media. Advisories are generally issued if a break in a water main has occurred, or the system has lost pressure. An advisory does not mean bacteria have been found in the water. This is a precautionary statement issued before water testing has been completed. A boil water advisory means a problem may have increased the risk for the water system to be contaminated. A boil water notice, on the other hand, is a notice to the public that tests show coliform bacteria are present in the water system.

Additional testing may take place and a water warning may also be released indicating fecal coliform bacteria are present. "Do not drink the water" notifications can be issued for either bacteria or chemical contaminants, which indicate that the water is so contaminated it should not be consumed, and boiling or disinfecting the water may not offer adequate protection.

Notifying Staff
After the organization learns its water supply has been contaminated, the following steps should immediately be implemented:
- The organization's Emergency Operations Plan (EOP) should go into effect, with consideration of opening the emergency operations center.
- Department leaders or their designees should meet in a predetermined place to await instructions from leadership about the incident.
- The public information officer (PIO) should draft a message for incident commander review and distribution, indicating a possible water contamination—additional instructions to follow.
- The incident commander should assign an individual to contact the local water department and/or water provider to determine the status of the incoming water.
- The logistics chief should reach out to water suppliers and place them on notice in the event water is required.
- After a determination is made about the water quality, the incident commander should brief leaders of the situation and outline a plan of response (*see* "Threat Analysis" on page 100.).

Cleaning the Organization
Nonpotable water may be used for cleaning work premises, other than food processing and preparation premises and personal service rooms[3] (rooms used for activities not directly connected with the production of service function performed by the establishment; such activities include, but are not limited to, first aid, medical services, dressing, showering, toilet use, washing, and eating). However, this nonpotable water must not contain concentrations of chemicals, fecal coliform, or other substances that could create unsanitary conditions or be harmful to employees.

Strategies health care organizations can use to keep facilities clean during a contaminated water emergency include the following:

- Keep it simple. General cleaning can be done in patient care areas using general disinfectant wipes commonly found in the organization.
- Consider premixed solutions. Many of the vendors supplying cleaning chemicals to the organization also have premixed chemicals available in their inventories. Keeping a small inventory of these supplies on hand could get the organization through a short-duration water emergency.
- Employ bottled or bulk potable water. Disaster plans often include a plan for responding to water emergencies that include a list of vendors that have already agreed to supply either bottled water for drinking or bulk potable water to the facility during a water emergency.
- Scale back. Leaders can curtail certain services or transfer patients to other facilities until the normal water supply to the organization has been restored. The organization should consider developing a water utilization list by department. The list would

(continued on page 104)

assist the incident commander in determining which process could be curtailed. The organization should consider developing a water utilization list by department. The list would assist the incident commander in determining which process could be curtailed.

Proper Preparation Is Key

Although water emergencies are relatively rare, they do occur and health care organizations must be ready to respond when they do. The Joint Commission standards require health care organizations to address the provision of water as part of the facility's EOP and prepare for how to manage utilities during an emergency. This includes identifying alternative water sources, and the organization implements the components of its EOP that require advance preparation to provide for utilities during an emergency. Proper planning also includes adding water emergencies into your hazard vulnerability analysis, particularly if your facility is located in a community where water emergencies often occur.

REFERENCES

1. Centers for Disease Control and Prevention. Emergency Water Supply Planning Guide for Hospitals and Health Care Facilities. 2012. Accessed Jun 24, 2016. http://www.cdc.gov/healthywater/pdf/emergency/emergency-water-supply-planning-guide.pdf.
2. LivingWaters™ Engineered Water Treatment Solutions. Contaminants. Accessed Jun 24, 2016. http://www.livingwatersway.com/water_contaminants.
3. US Occupational Safety and Health Administration. 29 CFR 1910, Subpart J: General Environmental Controls. [1910.141(b)(2)(iii).] Accessed Jun 24, 2016. https://www.osha.gov/pls/oshaweb/owadisp.show_document?p_table=STANDARDS&p_id=9790.

---

for creating a location for connecting the supplemental equipment. An example might be drilling a well for nonpotable water and placing the pump on emergency power to support toilet flushing on upper floors. A cutout on each floor could be used to access the hose to fill large 55-gallon trash containers with nonpotable water. Organizations should also establish with vendors the process for returning to normal operations.

An organization's EOP must address how the organization will deal with utilities failure—power; water; natural gas; medical gas; steam boiler equipment; heating, ventilating, and air-conditioning (HVAC); or other utility systems. The emergency response for utilities supporting general building function, medical equipment, and life safety may result in one or more of the following five broad categories of response.

Backup Systems

If the electricity supply fails, the facility will need to switch to backup generators and have the fuel to run them. These should be located on site in a secure manner, safe from unauthorized access or use, theft, and severe weather or other damage. There should be a supply of potable water and water for equipment accumulated on site as well. The organization should maintain medical gas supplies. In all cases, organizations should have considered how and be ready to integrate backup supplies into the normal systems. For instance, an organization could consider remote connections for additional emergency generators or water to continue to supply the minimum needs of the facility in the event of an emergency. If suppliers bring in supplementary water supplies, there must be a means for transferring that water from tanker trucks to the building water system and, if potable, testing to ensure that it is safe. Plans should be in place to instruct how to access safely stored extra fuel and also clarify how to make it easily accessible for vehicles during the emergency.

Repair and Replacement

If possible, malfunctioning primary systems should be repaired or replaced. Therefore, emergency managers need to plan for a supply of repair and replacement parts and equipment to be kept on site. If there is sufficient time before the onset of an emergency, they should also consider increasing staffing levels for clinical engineering, facility operations, and information management. Again, prearranged agreements with suppliers of repair supplies and replacement equipment will prove helpful in speeding up this process. For instance, during the hurricane season in Florida, generator mechanics will often be on site, sheltering with staff, to be available to help work through any problems with the equipment.

Alternative Means

If backup systems fail and equipment cannot be immediately repaired or replaced, the organization will need to implement its plan for reaching out to other sources to fulfill its needs. There may be equipment available that will prolong the organization's ability to provide services, but that may not be a long-term solution. The emergency management team in tandem with procurement may have to contact out-of-area suppliers to address shortages. They should keep contact information for likely sources in the incident command center. If the organization is part of a health care system, the parent entity of the affected facility may be able to provide supplies from other facilities it operates, according to prearranged agreements or policies. The organization may also be able to solicit supplemental supplies and equipment from community organizations such as fire departments, city or county government, state or federal emergency management assets, and so on.

Cessation of Services

Depending on the scope and duration of utilities failure, some or all of the services provided by the facility may have to be suspended or shut down. In the EOP, the emergency management team should identify who makes this decision, how and under what circumstances it is made, and how it is to be communicated to staff and outside entities. Leaders must notify The Joint Commission immediately if the organization must cease services, and they should be aware that cessation of services may impact the facility's accreditation status. (*See* Chapter 10 for a brief overview of the impact a cessation of services will have on accreditation status.)

Evacuation

In the case of a prolonged interruption of one or more essential utilities, the facility may need to be evacuated. Emergency planners will have planned for how the facility will be evacuated if, for instance, it has no electrical power. In the event that HVAC systems are down, staff may need to prioritize vulnerable populations in an evacuation. Staff leaders should practice evacuation procedures and post simulation debriefings to identify as many gaps and contingencies as possible. This also impacts the electronic medical record (EMR) and charting of patients.

Threat Analysis

Addressing a Utility Systems Failure

- Notify relevant staff and activate downtime procedures.
- Isolate and inspect affected systems.
- Communicate with backup source provider(s).
- Update leadership about repairs.
- Alert incident command staff to manage affected operations until systems restoration is achieved.

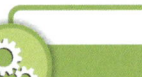

Capacity Builder

Utilities Failure Plan Checklist

Procedures for utilities failure will vary somewhat depending on which system fails, but there will also be a great deal of similarity. The following checklist may help you develop utilities failure and downtime/recovery procedures for each of your own critical systems:

Mitigation
- Identify and document who is in charge of maintaining the system and addressing failures (usually the engineering department).
- Identify and document the primary vendor.
- Identify and document the emergency vendor(s), if any.
- Identify who is responsible for testing and monitoring the system. Often this will involve working with the vendor. For example, water quality will generally be tested and monitored by local water authorities, with facilities monitoring delivery systems.

Preparedness
- Develop and follow standard procedures regarding the nature and frequency of testing and monitoring utilities.
- Drill for utility failures.

Response
- In response to system failure the engineering department will, if possible, isolate malfunctioning equipment, assess the extent of damage or failure, and commence needed repairs.
- Engineering staff will notify affected departments of the disruption.
- If applicable, engineering staff will notify the appropriate vendor or supplier of the outage.
- In the event of a widespread or facilitywide outage, the chief engineer or designee will inform facility administration.
- If necessary, engineering staff will inform organization staff of a widespread or prolonged disruption of service via mass notification systems such as overhead announcements using the appropriate code.
- In the event of a prolonged outage, initiate incident command and continuity of operations (COOP) to manage the outage and any existing supplies.
- Incident command notifies department heads to initiate departmental utility disruption procedures.

Recovery
- Consider the most efficient and timely recovery to normal operations as early in the process as possible, given the particulars of the disruption.
- Use facility and departmental business COOP plans to guide downtime and recovery efforts.

Source: Adapted from Kaiser Foundation Hospital Manteca/Modesto, Kaiser Permanente. [Systems Failure Plans.] California Hospital Association. Emergency Preparedness: Loss of Utilities/Systems. Accessed Jun 24, 2016. http://www.calhospitalprepare.org/loss-utilities-services.

Vulnerable Populations

Power Failure in Nursing Care Centers

Power loss presents a number of safety issues for residents of nursing care centers. Depending on the amount of time spent without power, residents who rely on the use of respirators and oxygen will undergo particular hardship. Although nursing care centers may have generators and backup batteries, it may not be enough to assist residents. The Emergency Operations Plan must make provisions, not only for utility loss, but also for the depletion of backup power sources. These plans can also address how loss of power may produce extreme temperatures within the facility. Residents may suffer illness due to heat stroke or cold exposure. Another safety concern for residents in a power outage might be its impact on automatic door locks or alarm systems. If these safeguards are rendered useless, and no contingency exists to replace them, residents could suffer injuries by roaming into areas that might pose risk to them such as stairwells, storage rooms, or even the kitchen area. They might even wander out of the nursing care center and become lost or harmed before staff became aware they are missing.

Because of the difficulty of moving and transporting geriatric residents, many of whom will need to be assisted or carried, sheltering in place is almost always the first choice of action, and evacuation should be considered only if the danger of staying outweighs the danger of moving so many vulnerable patients. Certainly, part of that calculation will depend on how long the outage is projected to last and whether the facility has adequate supplies to ride it out. Meals will need to be prepared. Linens will need to be washed or replaced. The operation of the facility, including delivery of medications and medical monitoring, will have to go on under backup power and lighting. Leaders will need to quickly assess the likely effects of the outage and determine how long they can stay in place. Then they can work with utility personnel to stay abreast of restoration efforts.

Effective management of supplies, solid planning for backup systems, and planning for backup systems failures will go a long way toward keeping facilities open and delivering care and services— even in extremely challenging situations. They will also ensure an orderly shutdown of the facility should that be necessary.

Recovery

It is absolutely imperative that the organization gets its facility back up and running normally as soon as possible after dealing with an emergency. To that end, the emergency management team should cultivate relationships with suppliers of utility equipment so that replacement and repair of the organization's utility equipment can be expedited to get the facility back on its feet after meeting the demands of an emergency situation.

Agreements with suppliers should be regularly tested and evaluated before and during exercises, as well as following actual responses, to assess how well they work during an emergency. And emergency planners will want to take into account the possibility that theirs might not be the only demands placed upon the services of their suppliers during and after an emergency. Other facilities may also need to replace or repair similar equipment. It's a good idea, therefore, to have a contingency plan in case a regular supplier is unable to provide goods and services in a timely fashion. (*See* Chapter 10 for a more in-depth look at recovery operations.)

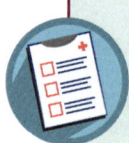

Case in Point
Sutter Medical Center in Sacramento Responds to a Loss of Backup Power

The Situation

Sutter Medical Center, Sacramento is the flagship hospital for Sutter Health, Northern California's largest health system. The hospital center consists of two acute care facilities connected seamlessly by a three-story spanning structure: the 242-bed Anderson Lucchetti Women's and Children's Center and the 281-bed Ose Adams Medical Pavilion. Early one morning, flooding in an underground vault knocked out an electrical switchboard, resulting in a loss of backup power to the Ose Adams Medical Pavilion, which houses the medical center's inpatient surgery and cardiac catheterization services.

Although primary power was not affected, without backup power, surgical and cath lab procedures could not be performed. Sutter is also home to large and busy adult and pediatric emergency departments (EDs). Because emergency patients often require surgery, the capacity of the ED to serve patients was severely compromised.

The Response

Within minutes the hospital command center was set up and emergency operations were initiated. The hospital's emergency management team began to work on a number of problems simultaneously:

Ambulances were diverted to other area hospitals while Sutter officials responded to the problem.

Within 30 minutes an alert was sent out to employees over the hospital alert system notifying them of the problem and soliciting help from managers.
- The team set out to find out how long it would take to repair the switchboard.
- They explored how long it would take to secure temporary backup power for the affected building.
- They looked into how the loss of backup power would affect hospital operations.
- They discussed how the loss of backup power would affect patients.
- They reviewed their Emergency Operations Plan procedures in case of a primary power failure to prepare for a double failure.
- They implemented a communications strategy to keep staff and the public apprised of developments.

It turned out that repairing the switchboard would take several weeks. The team decided to secure temporary backup generator power. By noon, semi-truck generators were on site, and electricians had them hooked up to the system and operational within 24 hours. In the meantime, surgical and ED staff began rescheduling elective surgeries and moving other surgery cases to the medical center's outpatient surgery facility and other operating rooms on the campus. In addition, surgical staff and managers took the opportunity to review evacuation procedures to prepare for safe movement of patients if the situation escalated.

Assessment and Conclusions

The flood presented a novel situation to the team. The affected vault and the equipment it contained had been in use for years, and it had never had a flooding problem before. However, over time water was allowed to seep into the vault and accumulate to the point where a failure occurred. In the wake of the incident the organization paid special attention to inspecting other such vaults for similar vulnerability.

The primary lessons learned from the incident were the importance of assembling a multidisciplinary team and of regular inspection and maintenance of utilities equipment. Sutter Medical Center, Sacramento's cross-disciplinary team of emergency managers, were able to convene quickly and work through several different aspects of the incident simultaneously. As a result, short- and long-term remedies could be initiated quickly, and operations at the facility could be modified in a way that allowed the organization to continue to deliver care such that most of its patients were not aware that anything out of the ordinary was happening that day.

IN SUMMARY

- Mitigation of utility system vulnerabilities should be a priority of capital investment.
- Thorough planning for utility system failure is essential because the health care organization cannot continue to deliver care for long without power, water, or gas.
- Prolonged utilities outages could lead to the need to evacuate. Organizations must plan for how to make an orderly exit, given the limitations imposed by, for instance, poor lighting, loss of climate control and refrigeration, loss of ventilation, loss of power, or lack of water.

CHAPTER 8

Caring for Patients

STANDARDS FOCUS

EM.02.01.01 The organization has an Emergency Operations Plan.

EM.02.02.11 As part of its Emergency Operations Plan, the organization prepares for how it will manage patients during emergencies.

AT A GLANCE
- Managing patient care
- Meeting patient needs
- Documenting information

WHO IS INVOLVED?
- Organization leaders
- Medical staff leaders, especially emergency department leadership
- Nursing leaders
- Support/ancillary staff
- Information managers
- Emergency manager
- Safety officer

Why Is This Critical?

The fundamental goal of emergency planning is to protect life and prevent injury. Patient care is the core mission of health care. During an emergency, patient care could be impacted by a surge in the number of patients (some of whom will need specialized care), severely limited resources, damage to the facility or its capabilities, or the need to evacuate the facility when it is no longer possible to provide care safely. Organizations must develop plans and procedures to meet the physical and psychological needs of patients. Their leaders need to document patient clinical and other information and to ensure that the information is transferred accurately to those who need it in a timely manner.

Key Planning Concepts for Patient Care

Certain clinical needs are so fundamental to providing and sustaining safe and effective care that organizations must have clear, reasonable plans to address those patient needs in extreme circumstances. A catastrophic emergency could result in a decision to keep all patients on the premises in the interest of safety. Conversely, it could result in the decision to evacuate the facility because it is no longer safe to stay. In either case, emergencies can disrupt everyday clinical processes such as admission, scheduling, and discharge, among others, and must be planned for as having a likely effect on patient care.

Decision Points

Health care facilities are often complex organizations engaged in a broad array of activities that cannot necessarily be stopped and started at a moment's notice. Part of the role of leaders is to identify those points in the progression of an emergency when critical decisions must be or can be made.

Initial Onset
The first decision point comes with the initial onset of emergency conditions or early notice that an emergency is likely or imminent. Some events are actually planned or predicted (for example, a known civic event such as the New York City Marathon or a visit by the president), and the health care organization may elect to open its emergency operations center and activate a portion of the Emergency Operations Plan (EOP) the morning of the known event. However, because most emergencies are by their nature unpredictable, conditions will continue to evolve as the situation unfolds. If a hurricane approaches, for example, at what point does a hospital or surgery center cancel elective surgeries? The severity of the emergency may increase, and the health care organization will decide at the point of notification or very shortly after to initiate its EOP.

Escalating Events
Secondary and tertiary emergencies (for example, an ice storm followed by a power failure) may increase the stress on the organization and its facilities and staff. Such emergencies are called escalating events; they compound the demands on the organization or degrade its capabilities to respond more rapidly. Ongoing monitoring of conditions and status is critical to maintaining situational awareness; when the situation changes significantly, as, for instance, if a fire or other internal emergency happens during disaster response, managers need to consider the possibility that the facility may need to curtail or cease operations and initiate an evacuation. Knowing when these decision points are likely to occur can help managers make decisions before the situation gets out of control.

Preparing for the Worst
Perhaps the most important decision that organization leaders and incident commanders must make is deciding if the facility will stay open during an emergency. Leaders must weigh the need for the organization's services during the emergency against the severity of the emergency's impact on the facility, including its ability to continue to deliver care and services while absorbing a potential patient surge (perhaps exacerbated by other health care organizations' inability to receive patients). Organization leaders and emergency managers should identify decision points at which the ability of the facility to continue to fulfill its mission, the risk to patients and staff, and other concerns can be evaluated. Sample decision points may include the following:
- Ability of other health care providers to absorb the patient load
- Role of the organization within the region—sole health care provider
- Facility damage assessment and duration of repairs
- Ability to obtain critical supplies: water, fuel, food, medical, pharmaceutical, staffing
- Patient acuity and ability to evacuate safely
- Environmental conditions

Patient Management
Disaster victims do not, by and large, arrive at empty facilities. They are transported to hospitals that are already in the full swing of normal operations with more or less normal patient loads. A potential surge of patients needing, for example, trauma care, decontamination, or isolation will put stress on staff and material resources, and the need to triage large numbers of incoming people will require appropriate staff, supplies, and space. Evaluating patients for early discharge to free bed spaces might be an option to consider in planning for patient surges.

Administration

To have enough space to triage and care for emergency patients in hospitals, it might be necessary to clear out the emergency department (ED) and/or inpatient beds and surge to overflow areas. The EOP should specify how to discharge patients who are able to go home. It should also define a process for identifying all the open beds in the facility, call for the immediate transfer of patients in the ED who require admission to inpatient beds, and outline the procedures for processing the remaining patients in the ED and others to arrive by ambulance or personal transport. Organizations might have to cancel elective surgeries to use operating room (OR) suites and free up personnel. Organization staff might also advise dialysis patients to go on specialized diets that make it possible for them to extend their wait for treatment.

In situations of patient surge, the EOP will define processes to support expedited triage and movement of patients through rapid treatment and discharge from the ED, or admission and in-house care. Where specialty needs exist that are not available at the hospital, the hospital will coordinate with coalition partners or community providers to obtain needed resources or transfer the patient as needed. Ancillary services such as radiology, laboratory, and pharmacy services are essential components of emergency planning and response for patient care. Support services such as transportation and housekeeping support efficiency in moving each patient through his or her phases of care. Administrative leaders should provide support to all units and services throughout the hospital to facilitate timely and effective scheduling, admissions, transfers, and discharges to help the organization accommodate a surge.

Triage

Organizations need to create and assess their triage plans and procedures ahead of time, and leaders need to work to make the triage system quicker and more effective by streamlining triage processes, making clear the expected flow of patients through triage to appropriate departments, and managing patients to create space in those departments sufficient to accommodate the surge.

Location, assessment, and treatment are among the major considerations for creating a fast, efficient, and effective emergency triage system. (*See* Figure 8-1 on page 116 for a sample protocol.)

Location

Large numbers of incoming casualties can quickly overwhelm the ED and its staff. The EOP should identify triggers for implementing emergency triage processes. Staff can set up triage stations in alternative areas of the facility that can be accessed by arriving emergency vehicles and that have access to the ED. If patients drive themselves or are driven by others, they may be able to reach the ED prior to ambulances. However, in the event of a possible infectious disease outbreak or radiological exposure, staff will need to separate incoming patients from the general population. By arranging triage outside of the facility (for example, in an adjacent parking lot or parking structure or a greenspace on the hospital campus), staff can direct potentially infectious patients to isolation. Those who require decontamination can be decontaminated before entering the facility.

Assessment

The use of triage questionnaires can speed up the process of sorting out those who need immediate attention from those whose needs are less pressing. This step can relieve strain on medical staff resources by allowing designated staff to perform the initial step in the triage process. The EOP should offer simple tools such as questionnaires and flowcharts that can show the patients' path through the triage system and also save time and resources in the process of educating staff.

In some instances, such as a radiological event, large numbers of physiologically unaffected people may present at the ED or triage station. Medical staff will need to quickly screen out those who are unlikely to have been exposed and direct them away from the facility and ED in particular. Staff need to ensure that critically ill patients are taken directly to the ED, even if they have not been decontaminated—there, they can be treated and stabilized prior to decontamination.

If the patients are triaged by emergency medical technicians during an event, they should arrive with a triage tag designation. The triage nurse will have to verify that the acuity of the patient has not changed during transport to the facility. Common triage tag colors include the following:
- Red —Critical/Major injuries
- Yellow—Moderate injuries
- Green—Minor injures
- Gray—Expectant (may not be able to survive)
- Black—Deceased

In a surge event, yellow and green tags will be given the highest priority, as the red tags may consume a significant amount of resources and have a lower survivability rate. Ethical considerations about which patients will receive what level of care should be reviewed by the organization's ethics committee.

Treatment

After staff assess a patient's need for care, they must determine where that patient needs to go to receive appropriate treatment and how that patient will get there. In particular, the EOP should account for how nonambulatory patients will move through the system and provide for equipment and staff to move them.

The organization may want to designate ahead of time areas of the facility to receive each category of triaged patient. Each area can then be staffed by personnel with appropriate skills and experience and stocked with supply carts containing appropriate equipment and supplies. For instance, licensed practical nurses (LPNs) could staff the area designated for the walking wounded, while ED and trauma care nurses would staff the area designated for the most urgent cases.

Evacuation

Senior organization leaders have a range of response strategies available to them, including closing service to new patients, internally evacuating one or more portions of the organization to another, and canceling certain services to make staff and medications available for other needs. When an organization's capabilities (staffing, facilities, supplies, and so forth) have been jeopardized to the extent that it will not be able to continue providing care safely, the decision to evacuate may be made. Prior to an emergency, organizations need to make detailed plans for how to evacuate patients safely and to drill staff on the implementation of those plans. Exercising how to evacuate different types of patients—such as intensive care unit patients, pediatric, morbidly obese, hearing or vision impaired, wheelchair bound—is essential so that staff can practice different challenges and be prepared to adjust their plans accordingly.

Evacuation is a complex process that requires advance coordination with receiving facilities and medical transport services, and often police and fire department authorities. It involves not only getting all patients out of the building but also the patient's clinical records, any specialized medication, supplies, and equipment they will need on the way, and, depending on the patient's condition, a staff member to accompany each individual patient to his or her receiving facility.

As discussed in Chapter 4, the emergency management team must keep a list of alternative care sites (internal and external) in the incident command post, including hospitals, nursing care centers, or other identified sites. It should contain contact information and information on the capacity and capabilities of each site. Staff will need to transport patients in need of intensive or specialized care to locations where that care is available. Noncritical patients and those not part of vulnerable populations have more flexibility in the kind of alternative care sites to which they may be transferred, or they may be discharged to home with follow-up through home care or their physician's office. And along with procedures for patient transfers, the EOP should describe the protocols for transferring medical records, care records, and other clinical information with each patient traveling to another clinical destination. Procedures also need to be in place to ensure the safe return of staff and medical equipment.

Meeting Patient Needs

In addition to medical needs, patients and other victims of a disaster will have other challenges that an EOP needs to address in planning for their care. These needs depend on the type of emergency, its scope, its duration, and the number of people requiring attention.

Hygiene and Sanitation

Some emergencies may cause disruption or limit access to normal sanitation and hygiene facilities. Organizations need to plan for this possibility by arranging for the deployment of portable toilets and the use of bedpans where appropriate. Plans should also account for how the waste will be stored and disposed of. Organizations can assess in advance what kinds of sanitation and hygiene activities (showering, hand washing, toilet use) will need to be accounted for by extrapolating from normal operational use.

Mental Health

In addition to addressing the physical health of patients, organizations facing emergency conditions must address the mental health of patients. During the emergency, organizations should consider patients' immediate mental health needs. This includes assessing needs quickly and frequently and providing crisis intervention or psychological first aid, utilizing behavioral health care consultation where necessary. Organizations can prepare for these needs by engaging in disaster behavioral health care planning and networking, specialized training initiatives for key staff, and community collaboration. During the transition from

Figure 8-1. **Sample Shelter Triage Form**

Shelter Triage Form

Contact Information				
Date:	Time:	Location:		
Name		Caregiver Name:		
Street Address:		Street Address:		
City:	State and Zip:	City:	State and zip:	
Age:	Sex:	Phone:	Cell:	

Acute Serious Illness			
Do you have pain, fever or any injury or illness which requires immediate medical attention?	NO↓	YES →	EMERGENCY ROOM
Are you dependent on a ventilator to breathe?	NO↓	YES →	Hospital or Nursing Home

Serious Medical Condition			
Do you receive home health nursing services?	NO↓	YES→	Medical Shelter
Do you have a contagious illness other than a cold?	NO↓	YES→	Medical Shelter
Are you have a suppressed immune system? (due to organ transplant, leukemia, current chemotherapy, current radiation therapy, other)	NO↓	YES→	Medical Shelter
Are you pregnant with a high risk pregnancy? (pregnant plus serious medical condition, or risk of loss of pregnancy or premature delivery)	NO↓	YES→	Medical Shelter
Are you in hospice?	NO↓	YES→	Medical Shelter
Do you need assistance with medication or glucose checks and no caregiver to assist, or have inadequate supplies?	NO↓	YES→	Medical Shelter
Do you have an open wound requiring dressing changes?	NO↓	YES→	Medical Shelter
Do you have seizures which are not under control?	NO↓	YES→	Medical Shelter
Are you on tube feedings?	NO↓	YES→	Medical Shelter
Are you bed bound?	NO↓	YES→	Medical Shelter
Do you have a central line, a tracheostomy, on oxygen, require bladder catheterization, require other special medical equipment or need daily IV meds?	NO↓	YES→	Medical Shelter
Do you have any other serious illness that would make care in a medical shelter necessary? If yes, specify:	NO↓	YES→	Medical Shelter

Figure 8-1. **Sample Shelter Triage Form** (continued)

Shelter Triage Form

	Support Needs			
Do you have a drug addiction which is not in remission (that is, to alcohol or any controlled substance)?		NO↓	YES→	Genpop with Support
Does the person have a mental illness which is not well controlled?		NO↓	YES→	Genpop with Support
Does the person exhibit problem behavior (e.g., due to confusion, memory impairment or cognitive disability)?		NO↓	YES→	Genpop with Support
Do you need assistance with activities of daily living (feeding, dressing, bathing, toileting) and have no full-time caregiver in the shelter?		NO↓	YES→	Genpop with Support
Are you unable to control your bowel or bladder?		NO↓	YES→	Genpop with Support
Do you need assistance with transfers and have no full time caregiver with you in the shelter?		NO↓	YES→	Genpop with Support
Do you need assistance due to sight or hearing impairment and have no full time caregiver or service animal with you in the shelter?		NO↓	YES→	Genpop with Support
Do you have a medical problem which prevents you from sleeping on a cot?		NO↓	YES→	Genpop with Support
Does the person have a cognitive impairment which will require them to receive assistance and have no full time caregiver?		NO↓	YES→	Genpop with Support
		General Shelter		

Figure 8-1 is a sample shelter triage form that organizations might use to identify the needs of their patients.

Source: North Dakota Department of Health. Shelter Triage Form. Jun 3, 2011. Accessed Jun 24, 2016. https://www.ndhealth.gov/flood/FORM%20-%20Shelter%20Triage.pdf. Used with permission.

Vulnerable Populations

Properly treating special needs populations during an emergency or disaster requires particular planning. As part of its EOP, an organization must plan to manage services for vulnerable populations served, including those who are pediatric, geriatric, or disabled, or have serious chronic conditions or addictions. In addition to those who are already in the facility when the emergency occurs, vulnerable populations, including those in the community and those receiving home care, might come into contact with the organization as the emergency develops. These populations may present special challenges with regard to managing specialized clinical needs, particularly if they have vison, communication, or mobility challenges requiring assistive support or equipment, or low English proficiency. The EOP and staff preparedness training should provide guidance and protocols for a number of vulnerable populations with a wide range of needs.

Pediatric Population

Children are included in this Joint Commission requirement because the differences between pediatric patients and the adult population are many and come into play in an emergency situation. For example, children cannot be decontaminated in decontamination units designed for adults. Young people are more vulnerable than adults to chemical agents that are absorbed through the skin or that are inhaled. They are also more susceptible than adults to dehydration, shock from biological agents, and radiation exposure.

Emergency department and unit staff should have the necessary training to treat these patients with the appropriate interventions in case of an emergency. Young children may not yet have developed the cognitive power to recognize some kinds of threats. Staff must be on the lookout for signs that indicate a physical threat to the children or to those who care for them. Because children also have unique psychological vulnerabilities, staff should be prepared to manage their particular needs in the event of mass casualties and evacuation.[1]

The American Academy of Pediatrics (AAP) recommends that hospitals incorporate into their emergency management planning "appropriate types and numbers of pediatric-trained staff, equipment, medications, and decontamination equipment, including the ability to handle nonambulatory children."[2](p. 563) In addition, the AAP says hospitals "must be prepared to handle situations in which patients will be cared for as a family unit and children will not be able to be separated from adults, such as in a quarantine situation."[2](p. 563) This requires hospitals to have the capability to care for children and for children's hospitals to be able to care for adult patients who would stay with their children. To ensure that these pediatric needs are adequately considered, hospitals should be sure to include pediatricians and emergency pediatricians in their emergency management planning, training, and drills.[2] Of course, ideally, wherever possible, health care coalitions and systems should plan for care at pediatric facilities for these patients.

Elderly Population

In long term care settings, the emphasis on disaster management is on the population served if it is an internal disaster. However, in a community emergency, the organization may be able to receive patients transferred from other inpatient or residential facilities, or may even have walk-ins. Every nursing care center must be prepared to effectively shelter in place, or to have preestablished relationships with other local nursing care centers to move residents from one facility to another, or—in the event of a community disaster—to safely transport residents to locations farther away. It could also mean that care is provided in austere care environments. This requires a systematic and redundant plan that takes into account individual needs, such as ensuring that patients' medication regimens are not disrupted in an emergency evacuation or that sensory aids such as eyeglasses, hearing aids, and so forth, are accounted for to minimize the patient's sense of disorientation.

Effective emergency management also depends on strong relationships among health care organizations and the community at large. Regional partnerships must be built and maintained to integrate planned responses before an emergency or a disaster occurs. This is particularly important when the emergency involves a special population such as the vulnerable elderly.

In the case of a communitywide emergency, all health care organizations might be needed—whether to assist with triage and urgent care of victims, provide nonurgent care to others, shelter community members or patients from facilities that have been evacuated, or supply specific staff and/or supplies to other organizations.

Special Needs Populations

In addition to children and the elderly, organizations may need to deliver care to other kinds of special or vulnerable populations—for example, those with limited proficiency in English, patients who live in institutional settings, patients with cognitive disorders or who may be developmentally delayed, patients with chronic medical conditions, or homeless people. To enhance the organization's ability to care for these patients, leaders may cultivate relationships with community-based agencies and organizations with more appropriate resources and greater experience dealing with these populations.

- Such external partners might include the following:
- Community health systems
- Faith communities serving diverse cultures
- Home health agencies
- Child care providers

Mitigating the Risk of Health Care Disparities

The Institute of Medicine, the American Hospital Association, the American Public Health Association, and many other organizations and associations have conducted research that finds that disparities in health care services in routine situations are often exacerbated during times of disaster.[3] When the health care organization serves vulnerable patient populations with limited English proficiency, or low-income communities (particularly black, Hispanic, and migrant communities), attention to equitable care and service during triage, assessment, treatment, discharge, or transfer can mitigate the risk of suboptimal care during response and excess demand for emergency and inpatient services during disaster recovery. Targeted emergency response strategies for diverse patient populations can include the following:

- Enlisting interpreter services where required
- Providing information and support to patient families around expedited discharges for care at home
- Drawing on community or coalition resources such as faith-based services and counselors to address psychological first aid needs and post-traumatic stress disorder

(continued on page 120)

> Diverse cultural groups know where their vulnerable neighbors live, are familiar with the strengths and resources in their communities, and can support health system resilience when they are engaged during response and recovery efforts.
>
> **REFERENCES**
>
> 1. Markenson D, Redlener I. Pediatric terrorism preparedness national guidelines and recommendations: Findings of an evidence-based consensus process. Biosecur Bioterror. 2004;2(4): 301–319.
> 2. Markenson D, Reynolds S; American Academy of Pediatrics Committee on Pediatric Emergency Medicine; Task Force on Terrorism. The pediatrician and disaster preparedness. Pediatrics. 2006 Feb;117(2): e340–362. Accessed Jun 24, 2016. http://pediatrics.aappublications.org/content/117/2/560.full.
> 3. Runkle, JD, et al. Secondary surge capacity: A framework for understanding long-term access to primary care for medically vulnerable populations in disaster recovery. Am J Public Health. 2012 Dec;102(12):e24–32. Accessed Jun 24, 2016. http://www.ncbi.nlm.nih.gov/pmc/articles/PMC3519329/.

response to recovery, organizations should plan for supportive counseling needs, screenings and referrals, support groups, and public education. (*See* "Setting Spotlight" on page 122 for more on addressing the mental health needs of patients and others who have experienced an emergency.

Mortuary Services

Unfortunately, the reality of emergencies is that some will result in an unusually high number of fatalities. The EOP needs to include a plan for mortuary services that will allow the organization to provide services in the event of a surge of fatalities. Organizations can keep a list of all morgues and mortuaries in their area, including emergency morgues, with contact and capacity information. The local city or county emergency preparedness program should include a plan to organize mortuary services in the event of a communitywide disaster. The organization's emergency manager should reach out to these local authorities to make sure that the organization's emergency mortuary services planning coordinates with that of the local community at large. In addition, organizations can identify surge capacity within their own facilities or at alternative care sites in case transport to off-site morgues or mortuaries becomes impractical or impossible. An example of good planning is working with the procurement team to identify refrigerated trailers that can be used to temporarily store bodies.

Planning should also extend to the provision of sufficient supplies such as body bags and tags and staff and vehicles for the transport of remains, special handling procedures for the remains of those who died from highly infectious disease, and tracking of casualties in the event that an unaccompanied patient is cared for at the hospital and loved ones contact the hospital to locate the deceased. Because road, weather, or other conditions could prevent vehicles from accessing the hospital for one to three days, the EOP should also include a morgue surge plan.

Documentation

Documenting and tracking patients' clinical information can be particularly challenging in an emergency situation because of increased patient volume, rapid transfers of patients, expedited patient management measures, the desire to provide care as quickly as possible to the largest number of people possible, and destruction or disabling of all or part of the medical record system.

Community Collaboration

Emotional Support

In times of crisis, it is important that first responders be trained by their organizations to identify and address the needs of people in the community impacted by the situation. This training should include knowing what signs to look for to identify people who need help in managing their emotions. Organizations can better prepare to help patients when they are able to assess their mental well-being. First responders can use these effective communication principles in making their initial mental health assessments[1]:

- Address people calmly and with warmth to put them at ease. This includes making eye contact and using a friendly tone.

- Build trust and help people to be comfortable enough to talk about their emotions. This includes making introductions and using a polite and respectful tone in asking questions.

- Explain the purpose of their questions, letting people know that there are no right or wrong answers.

- Listen. To truly help people, responders must show people respect and give full attention to their concerns.

REFERENCE:

1. US Department of Health and Human Services, Substance Abuse and Mental Health Services Administration. Psychological First Aid for First Responders: Tips for Emergency and Disaster Response Workers. Jan 2005. Accessed Jun 24, 2016. http://store.samhsa.gov/shin/content/NMH05-0210/NMH05-0210.pdf.

Documenting Patient Clinical Information

Limited resources, disruptions to utilities or communication, and a host of other issues that arise during an emergency add to the complexity of tracking critical patient information. Organizations could address these issues in a number of ways, such as using triage tags to identify the patient, the patient's condition, assessment, medications, and so forth. Documenting patient information might also be accomplished by using a paper medical record or a special abbreviated form of the record that has been created for emergency situations. Depending on the effect of the emergency on technology availability and use, organizations may also be able to document patient information through electronic medical records (EMRs). Documenting patient information is of primary importance; however, the emergency may impact the ability of organizations to keep clinical information current. The EOP must create contingencies for this potential problem.

Transferring Patients to Alternative Care Sites

Because space is limited, patients may be moving quickly through phases of care. They may be admitted, transferred, discharged, or transported to alternative care sites in a much shorter time frame than would happen under normal circumstances. So the EOP should describe the mechanisms by which clinical documentation can be transferred along with patients, whether by electronic transfer (if possible) or sending paper records along with each patient. (*See* Figures 8-2 and 8-3 for sample patient tracking forms.) The capacities of each receiving department or facility to staff the admissions area and to receive digital information are also concerns to be assessed and addressed in the plan.

Setting Spotlight

Behavioral Health Care

Anyone who experiences an emergency may need to seek out behavioral health care. An emergency's scope may impact a few individuals, or it may affect an entire population. Behavioral health care agencies need to address in an Emergency Operations Plan (EOP), how they will handle a wide spectrum of critical behavioral health care needs following a community disaster.

This will require coordinating with numerous entities that can help in the wake of an emergency. These agencies might include local law enforcement and fire departments, community counselors and pastoral staff, regional and state emergency medical services (EMS), the American Red Cross, and federal agencies.

Disaster response will begin with identifying who is in the most immediate need of on-the-scene mental health assistance and treat them first. Those treated may be victims, witnesses, bystanders, family and friends, or emergency responders. Assistance can be made available in churches, schools, various community centers and shelters, and similar sites. Care providers may include mental health professionals, substance abuse experts, social workers, psychologists, counselors, and clergy.

Crisis counselors will assess individuals' behaviors and emotional distress and will direct them to speak with care providers or agencies to help them work through the aftermath of the emergency. Easily perceived emotional symptoms such as anger, grief, confusion, and fear will identify many individuals needing help. Others, however, may be more difficult to read in terms of their stress levels and reactions to the situation. Behavioral health relief workers need to look for additional physical symptoms, such as fatigue, agitation, and self-isolation.

Tracking Patients

All of this rapid patient movement requires that the EOP account for the development of systems to track patients as they move through the environment of care and/or are transferred by staff to other facilities. Family members of patients may contact the facility to inquire about patients' well-being and whereabouts. Those queries need to be directed to a central location where such information is readily available.

For communication among clinicians, a real-time Web-based tracking system, such as the one adopted in New York State following Superstorm Sandy, could be used. That system tracks patients using scannable wristbands to deliver patient identity and clinical information to mobile devices. Organizations will need to have protocols in place to track unidentified patients—John or Jane Does. Their EOPs will need to include procedures for maintaining and entering clinical and other relevant patient information into the EMR system when it is back online.

Figure 8-2. **Sample Patient Tracking Form**

HICS 254 - DISASTER VICTIM/PATIENT TRACKING FORM

HOSPITAL INCIDENT COMMAND SYSTEM

1. INCIDENT NAME	2. DATE/TIME PREPARED	3. OPERATIONAL PERIOD DATE/TIME

4. TRIAGE AREAS (Immediate, Delayed, Expectant, Minor, Morgue)

MR#/ Triage #	Name	Sex	DOB/ Age	Area Triaged to	Location/Time of Diagnostic Procedures (x-ray, angio, CT, etc.)	Time sent to Surgery	Disposition (home, admit, morgue, transfer)	Time of Disposition

5. SUBMITTED BY	6. AREA ASSIGNED TO	7. DATE/TIME SUBMITTED

8. FACILITY NAME

Purpose: Account for victims of identified event seeking medical attention **Origination:** Situation Unit Leader
Copies to: Patient Registration Unit Leader and Medical Care Branch Director

HICS 254

Figure 8-2 provides a sample form organizations might use to track patients' conditions during an emergency.

Source: California Emergency Medical Services Authority. HICS 254—Disaster Victim/Patient Tracking. 2014. Accessed Jun 24, 2016. http://www.emsa.ca.gov/Media/default/HICS/Forms/HICS%20254-Disaster%20Victim%20Patient%20Tracking.pdf.

Figure 8-3. Sample Patient Evacuation Tracking Form

HICS 260 - PATIENT EVACUATION TRACKING FORM

1. Date	2. From (Unit)

3. Patient Name	4. DOB	5. Medical Record Number

6. Diagnosis	7. Admitting Physician

8. Family Notified ☐ YES ☐ NO NAME: _____ CONTACT INFORMATION: _____

9. Mode of Transport	10. Accompanying Equipment (check those that apply)		
☐ Hospital Bed ☐ Gurney ☐ Wheelchair ☐ Ambulatory ☐ Other:	☐ IV Pump(s) ☐ Oxygen ☐ Ventilator ☐ Chest Tube(s) ☐ Other:	☐ Isolette/Warmer ☐ Traction ☐ Monitor ☐ A-Line/Swan ☐ Other:	☐ Foley Catheter ☐ Halo-Device ☐ Cranial Bolt/Screw ☐ Intraosseous Device ☐ Other:

11. Special Needs

12. Isolation ☐ YES ☐ NO TYPE: _____ REASON: _____

13. Evacuating Clinical Location		14. Arriving Location	
ROOM # TIME		ROOM # TIME	
ID BAND CONFIRMED BY:	☐ YES ☐ NO	ID BAND CONFIRMED BY:	☐ YES ☐ NO
MEDICAL RECORD SENT	☐ YES ☐ NO	MEDICAL RECORD RECEIVED	☐ YES ☐ NO
BELONGINGS ☐ WITH PATIENT	☐ LEFT IN ROOM ☐ NONE	BELONGINGS RECEIVED	☐ YES ☐ NO
VALUABLES ☐ WITH PATIENT	☐ LEFT IN SAFE ☐ NONE	VALUABLES RECEIVED	☐ YES ☐ NO
MEDICATIONS ☐ WITH PATIENT	☐ LEFT ON UNIT ☐ PHARMACY	MEDICATIONS RECEIVED	☐ YES ☐ NO
PEDS / INFANTS		**PEDS / INFANTS**	
BAG/MASK WITH TUBING SENT	☐ YES ☐ NO	BAG/MASK W/ TUBING RCVD	☐ YES ☐ NO
BULB SYRINGE SENT	☐ YES ☐ NO	BULB SYRINGE RECEIVED	☐ YES ☐ NO

15. Transferring to another Facility / Location

TIME TO STAGING AREA _____ TIME DEPARTING TO RECEIVING FACILITY _____

Destination

TRANSPORTATION ☐ AMBULANCE. #____ AGENCY____ ☐ HELICOPTER ☐ OTHER

ID BAND CONFIRMED ☐ YES ☐ NO BY ____

DEPARTURE TIME: ____

16. Prepared by

PRINT NAME: _____ SIGNATURE: _____

DATE/TIME: _____ FACILITY: _____

HOSPITAL INCIDENT COMMAND SYSTEM

Purpose: Detail and account for patients transferred to another facility
Origination: Inpatient/Outpatient Unit Leader or Casualty Care Unit Leader
Copies to: Patient Tracking Manager, Medical Care Branch Director, evacuating clinical location, and Documentation Unit Leader

HICS 260 | Page 1 of 1

Print Reset Send Save

CHAPTER 8 | Caring for Patients

Figure 8-3. **Sample Patient Evacuation Tracking Form** (continued)

HICS 260 - PATIENT EVACUATION TRACKING FORM

PURPOSE: The HICS 260 - Patient Evacuation Tracking Form documents details and account for patients transferred to another facility.

ORIGINATION: Completed by the Operations Section as appropriate: the Inpatient Unit Leader, the Outpatient Unit Leader, or the Casualty Care Unit Leader, depending on where the identified patient is located.

COPIES TO: The original is kept with the patient through actual evacuation. Copies are distributed to the Patient Tracking Manager, the Medical Care Branch Director, the evacuating clinical location, and the Documentation Unit Leader.

NOTES: The information on this form may be used to complete HICS 255, Master Patient Evacuation Tracking Form. Additions or deletions may be made to the form to meet the organization's needs.

NUMBER	TITLE	INSTRUCTIONS
1	Date	Enter the date of the evacuation.
2	From	Enter the Unit the patient is leaving from.
3	Patient Name	Enter the patient's full name.
4	DOB	Enter the patient's date of birth (DOB).
5	Medical Record Number	Enter the patient's medical record number.
6	Diagnosis	Enter the primary diagnosis/diagnoses.
7	Admitting Physician	Enter the name of the patient's admitting physician.
8	Family Notified	Check yes or no; enter family contact information.
9	Mode of Transport	Identify mode of transportation needed.
10	Accompanying Equipment	Check appropriate boxes for any equipment being transferred with the patient.
11	Special Needs	Indicate if the patient has special needs, assistance, or requirements.
12	Isolation	Indicate if isolation is required, the type, and the reason.
13	Evacuating Clinical Location	Fill in information and check boxes to indicate originating room and what was sent with the patient (records, medications, and belongings).
14	Arriving Location	Fill in information and check boxes to indicate patient's arrival at the new location and whether materials sent with the patient were received.
15	Transferring to another Facility/Location	Document arrival and departure from the staging area, confirmation of ID band, and type of transportation used.
16	Prepared by	Enter the name and signature of the person preparing the form. Enter date (m/d/y), time prepared (24-hour clock), and facility.

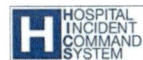

HICS 2014

Figure 8-3 provides a sample form organizations might use to track patients during an evacuation.

Source: California Emergency Medical Services Authority. HICS 260—Patient Evacuation Tracking Form. 2014. Accessed Jun 24, 2016. http://www.emsa.ca.gov/Media/default/HICS/Forms/HICS%20260-Patient%20Evacuation%20Tracking%20Form.pdf.

Reunification of Patients

The organization needs to have a process in place to ensure reunification during an emergency. It is likely that family members will become separated or that patients will be diverted to other health care facilities. Patients who are able to self-identify are the easiest to track. It's the patients who are not able to self-identify who become the challenge. Critical injuries, shock, or other medical issues may prevent a positive identification. Sample methods to identify patients include the following:

- Personal identification
- Check with the person who brought them in
- Photographs
- Community/school leaders (pastoral, teachers, and so forth)
- Fingerprinting—requires assistance of law enforcement

> **Case in Point**
> **A Hawaiian Hospital's Response to an Earthquake**
>
> At 7:07 a.m. on Sunday, October 15, 2006, the ground began to shake violently on the Big Island of Hawaii. For the next 40 seconds, a 6.7 magnitude earthquake turned a peaceful morning upside-down at Kona Community Hospital, a 94-bed facility in Kealakekua, Hawaii.
>
> **Making the Decision to Evacuate**
> There were 69 patients in the hospital at the time the earthquake hit. The 40-second event rendered the hospital's long term care unit, medical/surgical unit, obstetrics (OB) department, and two of three operating rooms (ORs) unsafe for patient care. No patients or staff members were harmed during the earthquake; however, by the time the CEO arrived on site at the hospital, a night supervisor had already made the decision to evacuate the previously mentioned areas based on their condition. The evacuation went smoothly, and no staff or patients were injured during the process. The provision of care was never interrupted. Kona's staff was well prepared for the evacuation procedure because the hospital has a disaster plan that covers potential evacuations that is exercised twice a year.
>
> Despite the damage to certain areas of the hospital, the intensive care unit (ICU) and emergency department were undamaged. With the potential of receiving an influx of emergency patients from earthquake-generated destruction, the hospital made the decision to keep those two departments open. In addition, the hospital's inpatient psychiatric unit suffered mild damage but did not have to be evacuated.
>
> **Moving Patients Outside**
> During the evacuation, patients were moved to several different areas. An OB patient in active labor was moved to the ICU, where she delivered a healthy baby later that day. The acute care patients from the medical/surgical unit were moved into a tent outside, and when that tent filled up, the organization moved patients under trees to take advantage of the shade. The hospital's 29 long term care residents were moved to shaded areas along the rear parking area of the hospital. Staff and supplies went with all the patients, and bedridden patients went outside in their beds. While moving everyone outside to covered areas was an initial response, it was untenable to leave patients

outside for too long. The sun in Hawaii is very intense, and sunburn and dehydration were potential threats to patients' health and safety.

Finding Alternate Sites

The county civil defense plan identified a community meeting center as an evacuation site for the hospital's patients, but the earthquake had rendered that facility without power or air-conditioning, and there was no backup generator for the site. The center was not viable for patient and staff use. Moving people back into the hospital wasn't an option, so staff had to come up with alternatives.

The Administrative Services Building across the driveway from the main portion of the hospital has two large classrooms on the lower level. After a quick assessment of the building, it was determined that although the upper level was damaged, the lower level was not and could accommodate the displaced patients. Hospital staff and civil defense volunteers moved classroom contents into nearby hallways and offices and cleaned the classrooms. All the medical/surgical patients—along with their beds, supplies, and staff—were moved to this location, where the hospital was able to provide care.

By the end of the day, all patients who required continued hospitalization were flown to Hilo Medical Center, located on the east side of the Big Island. Kona and Hilo are part of Hawaii Health Systems Corporation's network of hospitals that exists throughout the Hawaiian Islands. They have standing protocols to help each other however they can. Hilo Medical Center is at least two hours away from Kona Community Hospital—if the traffic isn't bad and the roads are open; however, the earthquake made driving to Hilo out of the question.

Getting patients to Hilo Medical Center was a community effort. Ground transportation to the airport was provided by a local ambulance service. The Coast Guard provided a Disaster Medical Assistance Team along with a C-130 transport aircraft.

Kona's long term care patients were temporarily housed in the conference area of a local resort after the local fire chief had contacted the Sheraton Keauhou Bay Resort, and they agreed to help. Spearheaded by the facilities director, the hospital moved the 29 residents, their beds, and other equipment—including a medication dispensing unit—the nine miles to the resort. Wheelchair-bound residents were moved in the hospital's handicapped-accessible van, and a local tour bus company made buses available to move the ambulatory residents. In addition, a local trucking company provided trucks and staff to help move the beds, tables, and other equipment the residents were going to need.

Establishing Relationships Before an Emergency

Prior to the earthquake, Kona Community Hospital had established a relationship with its community's emergency responders, including fire, police, county, and Coast Guard officials. One of the organization's annual emergency management exercises coordinates activities with other community agencies. This exercise familiarized the hospital with the capabilities of the community's disaster preparedness system. The CEO credits this collaboration with the success of the hospital's evacuation.

IN SUMMARY

- Decide early whether to activate the EOP as it relates to patient care and maintain situational awareness so that patient care plans can be adapted to changes in the environment of care or availability of appropriate space, supplies, and staff.

- Continue to monitor resources and the ability of the organization to deliver care, and set specific indicators and triggers and key decision points, including when evacuation should be initiated.

- Consider the challenges posed during emergency care and evacuation for special or vulnerable populations, such as the elderly, pediatric patients, midsurgery patients, or mental and behavioral health patients.

- Include procedures in the EOP for tracking evacuated patients and ensuring their safe transport and continued care in the event of an evacuation.

CHAPTER 9

A Framework for Testing and Evaluation

STANDARDS FOCUS

- **EM.02.01.01** The organization has an Emergency Operations Plan.
- **EM.03.01.01** The organization evaluates the effectiveness of its emergency management planning activities.
- **EM.03.01.03** The organization evaluates the effectiveness of its Emergency Operations Plan.
- **LD.04.04.01** Leaders establish priorities for performance improvement.

AT A GLANCE

- Analyzing and reviewing the hazard vulnerability analysis, objectives and scope of the Emergency Operations Plan (EOP), and inventory annually
- Designing emergency exercises
- Implementing and monitoring implementation
- Evaluating emergency exercises
- Improving preparedness and the EOP

WHO IS INVOLVED?

- Organizational leadership and clinical leadership should develop tools and design exercises to help evaluate preparedness, but everyone should be involved in the process of evaluation and testing.

Why Is This Critical?

Testing and evaluation of the Emergency Operations Plan (EOP) is essential both because it keeps staff familiar with emergency operations procedures and their roles in an emergency, and because it is an opportunity to assess the strengths and weaknesses of planning and preparedness and to further support incident command structure training for new staff and staff in different supporting roles.

Key Concepts for Testing and Evaluation

Exercises offer a way to assess the adequacy and appropriateness of response, logistics, human resources, and training. It is where the EOP moves from concept to reality. Because the nature of threats is constantly evolving, and because organizations are also constantly evolving, a continuous process of exercises, evaluation, and modification of the EOP is essential. The Joint Commission standards mandate that organizations implement the EOP at least twice annually in most settings, through exercises or actual responses, so this process should be recursive and ongoing.

During an emergency or planned exercise, the organization must carefully monitor the six critical areas of emergency management—communications, resources and assets, safety and security, staff responsibilities, utilities, and patient clinical and support activities. These functions are essential to providing care and protecting patients and staff. Exercises should be sufficiently robust to stress the system and test leadership decision making and contingency planning during the dynamics of the event. In addition, exercises provide staff the opportunity to practice providing care using modifications in clinical or administrative processes, in altered communication procedures, and with different equipment, supplies, team members, or locations.

Planning Evaluation Activities

While The Joint Commission requires organizations to test their EOPs by activating them for exercises or actual responses at least twice annually, freestanding buildings classified as business occupancy that are not designated community disaster receiving sites need to activate their EOPs only once per year. For facilities that provide emergency services or are designated community disaster receiving stations, at least one exercise per year must involve an influx of actual or simulated patients. The timing of these exercises is up to the organization, but the organization must demonstrate that it has integrated improvements, revisions, or lessons learned from the previous exercise into the subsequent exercises. It is also a good idea to vary the time of day and the day of the week on which the exercises will be held to make sure that the maximum number of staff is brought into the emergency planning process and the widest array of circumstances may be considered.

Types of Exercises

There are four major types of emergency exercises.

Drills

Drills are designed to test individual facets of the organization's response capabilities so that emergency planners can evaluate individual parts of the EOP. Commonly, they are narrowly focused, often confined to one department or a small number of related departments.

Tabletop Exercises

A tabletop exercise involves key personnel discussing simulated scenarios and is used to assess plans, policies, and procedures. It is a discussion-based exercise that familiarizes participants with current plans, policies, agreements, and procedures, or may also be used to develop new plans, policies, agreements, and procedures. Tabletop exercises are not sufficient to fulfill the exercise requirement (except for certain home care settings using defined criteria), but they are valuable tools for working through components of emergency response as a team.

Functional Exercises

A functional exercise is a simulated disaster designed to test the organization's actual response. A functional exercise validates the coordination of the emergency response activities within the organization, including collaboration with planning and response partners. It is an operations-based exercise that is action-oriented and designed to validate plans, policies, agreements, and procedures; clarify roles and responsibilities; and identify resource gaps in an operational environment.

Full-Scale Community Exercises

These are comprehensive, communitywide tests of emergency response that help the health care organization's emergency planners evaluate the organization's ability to work within the wider community response framework. These exercises are typically not designed by the organization, but by the local or regional emergency operations center. To the extent that the health care organization has a role in community emergency response, it will be expected to participate in relevant drills and exercises; this participation can count toward the organization's Joint Commission exercise requirement.

Patient Influx

Because mass-casualty events can generate hundreds of victims in a community, some exercises should have a component that reflects such scenarios and simulate the challenges

---

Capacity Builder

Exercise Planning

- What will the emergency be? This should be as specific as possible to offer the most realistic test of the plan. For example, a mock disaster involving bioterrorism should be specific, as clinical treatments vary, depending on the problem.
- What are the goals and objectives of the exercise? There should be general goals, but also specific subgoals or targets that help gauge success of processes and outcomes—for example, triage of 100 patients in one hour, clearing 6 emergency department (ED) beds in 15 minutes, decontaminating 10 special-needs patients each hour. How are the goals tied to the six critical areas?
- Which departments in the organization will be involved? For example, it makes sense to go beyond the ED in a hospital, or clinical care areas in a nursing care facility, to reach into other areas that would be called on during an emergency. For example, will pharmacy or the laboratory be included?
- Will the exercise run across multiple shifts?
- How can the exercise be conducted without disrupting normal care provided?
- How will patients and the community be made aware of the exercise so that it is not mistaken for a real crisis?
- How can the exercise be made scalable? In other words, how can components be added to or deleted from the exercise scenario to make it more complex and demanding (that is, escalated) or less so?
- What supplies and equipment will be included in the exercise?
- How will communication, including the effectiveness of communication both within the organization and with those in the community, be maintained and monitored?
- What provisions will need to be made for safety and security, both as part of the planned exercise and to maintain normal operations?
- How is the exercise related to the hazard vulnerability analysis?
- Will the exercise be announced or unannounced to staff?
- Will the emergency operations center be opened?
- How and when will the exercise end? Will it be completed at a certain time of day or when a particular outcome is achieved?

that accompany a surge of individuals seeking care. Procedures that could be tested in relevant exercises include the organization's plans for the following:
- Triaging 100 patients an hour within limited space with staff on hand
- Isolating infectious patients using dedicated teams in a newly constructed space
- Decontaminating dozens of injured patients exposed to an unidentified chemical agent
- Replenishing pharmaceuticals through requests to the state's emergency operations center
- Confirming the supply chain for food for 100 additional patients plus supporting staff with families for a projected six-day weather disaster

Scaling/Escalating the Response

Organizations should consider running exercises that simulate multiple emergencies to test the organization's resiliency and assess the ability of staff to change tactics as the situation changes or escalates. Simulation of a slowly evolving situation will test the organization and its staff in different ways than simulation of a quickly evolving one. Similarly, tactics will change with variations in complexity. For example, a tornado creates a path of destruction resulting in a mass casualty situation. As the patients begin to arrive, power is lost, requiring the organization to go on emergency power. This may seem like a manageable exercise, but now factor in an upset family member brandishing a weapon, media gaining access to patients on the inpatient unit, and closure of the main access road to the organization. Real events normally have multiple emergencies that will test the ability of the organization to operate.

Stand-Alone Response

Organizations are required to conduct at least one exercise a year that is escalated so that the organization can determine how it will cope without the support of the local community. Conducting exercises involving multiple elements of an emergency at one time, such as a large influx of patients and a simultaneous loss of power, makes the drill more challenging. Unless the exercise stresses the system, it will not provide insight into strengths and weaknesses.

For example, an exercise might require adapting rapidly to different supplies or equipment, or it might drain on-hand inventory to test organization processes for obtaining more equipment, medical supplies, pharmaceuticals, food, water, linens, staff, and so forth. Exercises should push participants to explore existing agreements with suppliers and to activate contingency plans when primary agreements fall through. For example, the organization might have a designated individual call vendors to explain that an exercise is in progress and to ask how long it would take to deliver the supplies. This tests the ability to reach suppliers and see how quickly they can deliver the needed supplies and equipment.

Those designing the exercise may consider including vendors in the exercise scenario (for example, by having them work through logistical problems during the exercise, such as the inability to deliver supplies due to serious weather or problems of scarcity, or as in the event of several health care organizations requesting help simultaneously). The exercise should also push staff to problem-solve outside of their familiar routines and without their usual resources.

Communitywide Exercises

At least once a year, the organization must participate in an emergency exercise involving a communitywide disaster response to evaluate areas of the EOP that deal with large-scale disasters and coordination and collaboration with outside agencies, such as health system response partners, public health authorities, emergency medical services, fire department, police department, local businesses, and volunteer patients. Alternative care sites should be included because testing increases communitywide awareness of the existence, location, strengths, and challenges of such facilities. It also encourages face-to-face interactions so that responders become familiar with one another.

Many state health departments and state hospital associations sponsor annual statewide or regional disaster preparedness exercises that reflect key clinical and operational elements required in accreditation standards. Health care organizations can investigate which federal, state, or local emergency exercises, such as Urban Shield, will be taking place in their area in which they might participate.

Monitoring Response

Having observers on hand to monitor response activities during emergency exercises will enhance the organization's ability to evaluate these activities later. It is a good idea to designate at least one person whose sole duty during the exercise is to observe and monitor the response. If possible, multiple observers should be assigned, be they staff or outside observers with a background in health care emergency management or related fields. Observers should document the performance of emergency system procedures; coverage of the six critical areas as relevant to the emergency scenarios; staff use of expected protocols, equipment, and supplies; safety and security of the participants; staff use of communication channels or of improvised strategies where needed; and so on.

Evaluating Exercises and Actual Responses

For an exercise or actual response to be of value in refining emergency management and response, it is essential that the organization be able to evaluate its performance. Typically, this process involves compiling the contents of after-action reports by participants and observers, performance data, and other information, using that information to identify areas in which the organization did not meet the desired standard of performance, and analyzing it to try to understand why.

The compiled data and reporting can then be analyzed in order to identify deficiencies and areas for improvement to policies, procedures, and performance. After deficiencies in response are identified, the organization can prioritize preparedness improvements intended to address those deficiencies, and make any necessary modifications to the EOP. The goal of subsequent exercises is then not only to identify further areas for improvement but also to assess whether the previous prioritized improvements in preparedness are having the desired effect.

Case in Point
Communitywide Emergency Response Exercise and Operating Room Evacuation Drill

Beth Israel Deaconess Medical Center (BIDMC), located in Boston and affiliated with Harvard Medical School, is one of the foremost teaching hospitals in the United States and a national leader in education, research, and technology. BIDMC has more than 1,200 physicians on its active medical staff (including more than 800 full-time staff physicians), most of whom hold faculty appointments at Harvard Medical School. In addition to a full range of clinical services, from neonatal intensive care to cancer treatment to transplant surgery, BIDMC is an industry leader in safety and security.

On May 3, 2014, BIDMC participated in Urban Shield: Boston, a communitywide federal emergency response exercise. Urban Shield is primarily designed to assess the response of first responders to complex public safety situations. However, area hospitals are called upon to participate in some of the scenarios to assess both their own emergency response and the quality of their coordination and cooperation with other responding agencies. In this case, area hospitals simulated a full evacuation of Massachusetts General Hospital, an event that forced all surrounding hospitals to accommodate a substantial patient surge in the midst of the disruption caused by multiple emergencies in the area and the response to them. But emergency planners at BIDMC wanted to go deeper and test their response beyond the general level. Accordingly, to assess the staff and the organization's ability to provide care to special populations during an emergency, that afternoon BIDMC staged a lockdown and evacuation drill coving seven in-use operating rooms.

Scenario and Setup

The scenario for the drill involved a bomb detonating in a parking deck beneath a bridge that joins two operating room pods, with three operating rooms on one side and four on the other. The exercise was conducted on a Saturday, both to coincide with Urban Shield and because the operating rooms would normally be vacant at that time. Medical students were brought in to play the roles of patients. Seven surgery teams were brought in, and each was given a patient scenario when the exercise began that provided details about the patient, the patient's condition, what surgery was being performed, how far the procedure had progressed, and the current status.

The surgery teams were given the following goals:
- Stabilize the patient for evacuation.
- Immediately evacuate horizontally to the postanesthesia care unit (PACU) and await instructions.
- If necessary, evacuate vertically, and prepare patients for transfer to other facilities.

To add complexity, after the drill was initiated, the area of the hospital including the surgical pods was placed on security lockdown, some areas were designated as structurally damaged and impassible, hallways were dressed with black and gray streamers to signify smoke, and the fire alarm was triggered. Observers were posted throughout the units and along the evacuation route to observe and assess performance and to ensure that the teams adhered to all the normal rules governing the movement and evacuation of surgical patients.

Response

According to Meg Femino, director of emergency management at BIDMC's Silverman Institute for Health Care Quality and Safety, the surgical teams succeeded in stabilizing their patients and evacuating the operating rooms in approximately four minutes. Once in the PACU, teams were directed to evacuate their patients down the stairs to the emergency department for further stabilization and transfer to other hospitals. This evacuation was accomplished by carrying the patients, complete with mock ventilation tubes and intravenous (IV) apparatus, down the stairs on evacuation sleds.

Assessment and Conclusions

After-action reports were solicited from all participants and observers, and a comprehensive assessment was compiled. Femino reports that the response was generally very good. The evacuation from operating rooms was speedy, the surgeons turned evacuation procedures over to the nursing staff as the transition was made from horizontal to vertical evacuation, and a well-drilled nursing staff effected a fast and safe transport of the patients down the stairwell to the emergency department. However, several areas for improvement were identified in the reports. Operating room staff and PACU staff did not seem to know each other's strengths and weaknesses, which hampered their ability to work together. This may have been symptomatic of a broader problem. Though the surgeons did an admirable job of leading the teams through the horizontal evacuation and passing off responsibility to the nursing staff, it was unclear who was ultimately in charge from that point forward, and this led to some confusion and miscommunication. In addition, some staff seemed unfamiliar with the two-way radios used for emergency communication, highlighting the need for further training.

Femino credits the culture of teamwork and team responsibility for the positive aspects of performance, noting that although some federal money was allocated to pay participants for coming in on a weekend for the exercise, the physicians did this on their own time. BIDMC tries to run full-scale exercises like these at least every four to five years, with more limited exercises at least twice annually. Nursing teams drill with their evacuation sleds during nursing competency days. These exercises not only keep emergency procedure skills sharp among the staff, they help the staff cultivate personal working relationships across departments and teams that facilitate better emergency response. (*See* Figure 9-1 for a helpful matrix emergency planners at BIDMC use to plan their drill scenarios.)

Figure 9-1. Planning Matrix

	Documents	Description	Status	Complete (Y/N)
Emergency Management: Drill Planning Matrix				
Drill Name:				
Drill Date(s):				
Planning Committee:				
Objectives	Objective Matrix	List of each department/critical area within the drill and the objectives relating to each one		
Scope/ Scenario	Drill Summary Document	Scenario, players, goals		
	Executive Summary Document	Detailed summary of the drill, critical tasks that will be performed, basic events list		
Pre-Planning	Save the Date(s)	Brief description of the drill, with date(s) and location included		
	Photographer (if needed)	Schedule with Media Services.		
	Book Venue	Coordinate with EM Admin.		
Resources	Resource/Equipment List	List of all equipment/resources needed to execute the drill efficiently (e.g., extra linen, decon tent, dashboards)		
	Patient Scripts / Patient Master List (if needed)	If the drill involves simulated or volunteer patients, create scripts & a corresponding master list.		
Drill Materials	Master Exercise Scenario List (MESL)	A spreadsheet containing each critical component of the scenario and "expected" response by specific departments, organized sequentially		
	Rules of Play Document	All of the standard rules of play for a drill		
	Sign-In Sheets			
	Evaluation Forms	Given to drill evaluators, listing each objective and/or critical task expected to occur during the exercise		
Volunteers	Instruction Document	Contains what volunteers can expect to happen during the drill, location, time(s), and basic logistics		
	Permission Slip (if needed)	Needed especially if there is off-site travel needed		
	Photo Waiver (if needed)	Needs to be signed by volunteer and/or parent to be allowed to photograph the drill		
After Action/Final Actions	After-Action Report	Utilize BIDMC EM AAR template. Once complete, ensure items are added to AA Matrix/ Performance Metric.		

EM, Emergency Management; BIDMC, Beth Israel Deaconess Medical Center; AAR, After-Action Report; AA, After Action.

Figure 9-1 provides guidelines to evaluate areas of emergency preparedness during planning exercises.

Source: Adapted from Femino M. Drill Planning Matrix. Beth Israel Deaconess Medical Center, Boston. Used with permission.

Multidisciplinary Process

Evaluation of exercises and actual responses should be a multidisciplinary collaboration that brings together quantitative and qualitative feedback provided by participants, volunteers, observers, and managers. Direct observation by observers or managers of the performance of frontline department staff can help managers and emergency planners understand the challenges faced by those delivering care in emergencies, but it is at least equally critical that managers be open to the upward flow of information from ground-level staff. Staff participating in an exercise or actual emergency response should be fully debriefed. They should be encouraged to share their accounts of the experience, their opinions about what went right and what went wrong, and quantitative evaluations of emergency response in their departments. Leaders can expect honest feedback when they offer staff opportunities for open discussion without fear of recrimination.

Community Collaboration

Coalition Exercises

Health care coalitions are a coalition of health care, community, and regional organizations. Mutual Aid Coordinating Entity (MACE) is an example of a coalition in the Hudson Valley region that understands the value of supporting one another. Members of the coalition have agreements in place to assist each other and pool efforts and resources in emergency situations. However, that is not the only time they work together. They prepare for this partnership by participating in shared exercises and simulations.

One such exercise, held in conjunction with Westchester County Airport, is a simulated plane crash, held to meet the requirements of the Federal Aviation Administration (FAA). The participants in the exercise included a number of emergency management agencies, the police department, multiple fire departments, several major airlines, and volunteers from the community. The emergency exercise consisted of emergency responders quickly attaining available bed counts from county hospitals and then working with their community partners in transporting "victims" from the scene. The airport conducts and improves upon this exercise every two years.

MACE also participated in a National Disaster Medical System (NDMS) exercise in conjunction with Stewart Air National Guard Base. This exercise is designed to test the response capabilities of medical organizations in emergency scenarios. In this instance, participants coordinated the removal of over a hundred volunteer "patients" from military transport planes and transported these casualty victims from a "war zone" to providers of care.

As all participants in these exercises would concur, repeated trainings such as these are the best way to gauge preparedness and to make improvements in response (*see* Figure 9-2 on page 138 for a drill planning guide to use when conducting exercises).

Figure 9-2. Emergency Management: Exercise Planning Guide

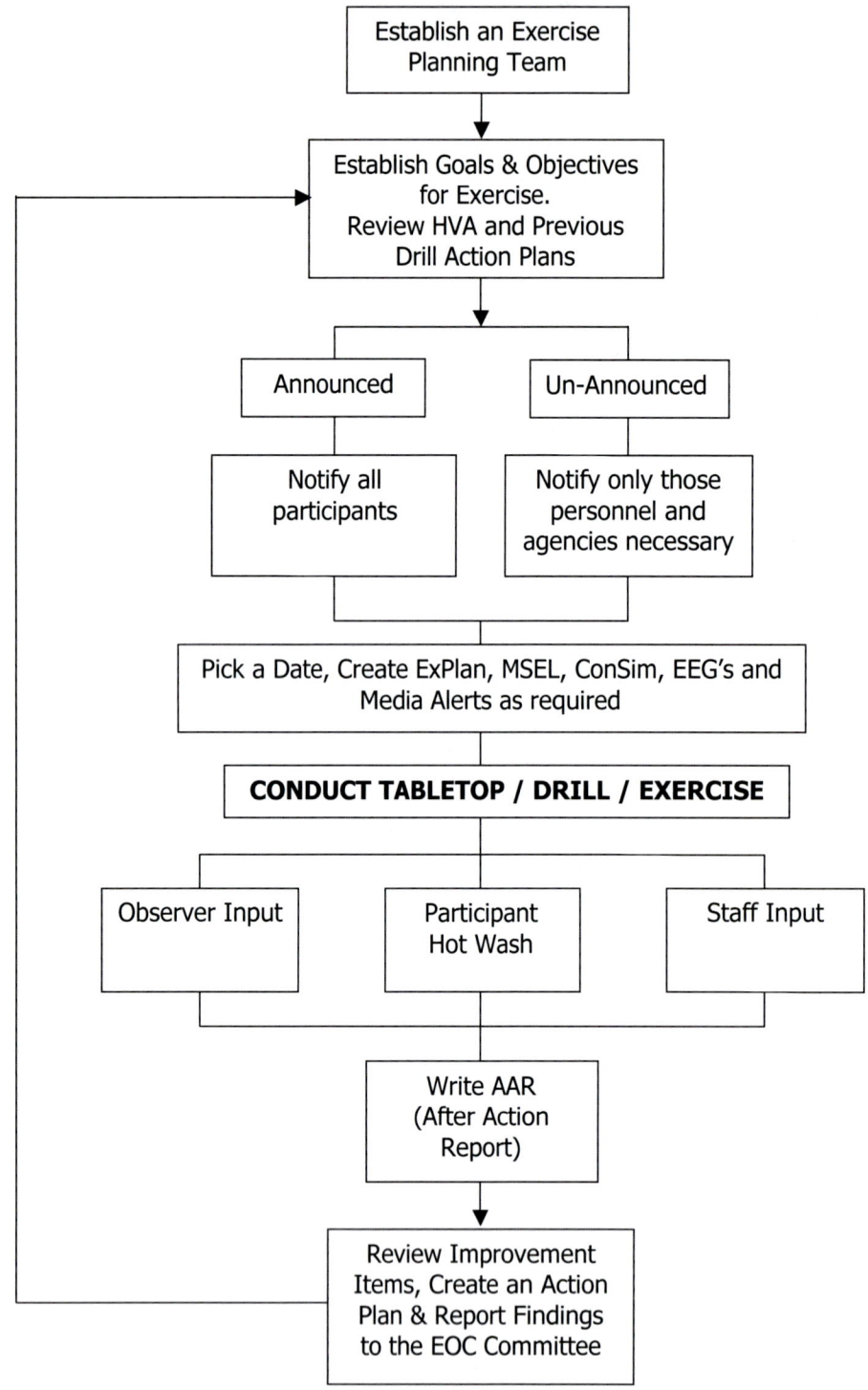

HVA, hazard vulnerability analysis; ExPlan, Exercise Plan; MSEL, Master Scenario Event List; ConSim, Control Simulator; EEG, Exercise Evaluation Guide; EOC, Environment of Care.

Figure 9-2 illustrates the process flow of emergency exercise planning.

Source: Adapted from Tangredi E. Emergency Management: Exercise Planning Guide. White Plains Hospital, White Plains, NY. Used with permission.

Case in Point
University of Nebraska Medical Center/Nebraska Medicine's Biocontainment Unit Uses a Collaborative Model to Treat Patients Infected with Ebola Virus Disease

Planning and Preparation

From discussions beginning in 2002 about ways to treat patients with highly infectious diseases while minimizing the risk of infection to staff, health care workers, and the community at large, a collaboration was born between the University of Nebraska Medical Center, Nebraska Medicine (the hospital), and the Nebraska Department of Health and Human Services. In 2005 this collaboration resulted in the opening of the Nebraska Biocontainment Unit (NBU) on the campus of the University of Nebraska Medical Center. The NBU is a 10-bed facility specifically designed and staffed to meet the challenges of treating patients with highly infectious diseases.

Because the transport, housing, and treatment of these highly infectious disease patients requires special policies and procedures in almost every aspect of care, NBU leadership assembled a cross-disciplinary, highly specialized team from among the health system staff to handle issues ranging from safe transport to infection control to waste management to finance and procurement. When activated, the NBU team is managed under the Hospital Incident Command System (HICS) structure and stresses coordination and communication. This kind of communication is critical in an environment in which error in protocol or a gap in procedure can require a lifesaving intervention. And, in fact, many NBU staff have cross-disciplinary backgrounds themselves, which further facilitates interprofessional collaboration in both training and practice.

The unit would be activated in September, October, and November 2014 to care for three Americans, two of whom were health care workers, who had contracted Ebola Virus Disease (EVD) while working in western Africa. Prior to that, NBU leadership and staff engaged in a variety of drills and exercises with several main goals. First, the drills were intended to develop and maintain competencies among the staff in the particular procedures, protocols, and policies involved in treating patients with highly infectious diseases, including an all-hazards planning approach that took into account complicating factors such as the possibility of severe weather and other challenges. Second, exercises allowed NBU staff to assess the adequacy and efficacy of policies and procedures with an eye toward continuous refinement and improvement. Third, the NBU was used as a laboratory for the study of infectious disease care where researchers could study and develop best practices for personal protective equipment (PPE) protocols, ventilation design, waste management, morgue procedures, and a host of other issues. Finally, the drills enabled the staff to become familiar with each other, developing a trust that facilitated future teamwork.

By the time the first EVD patient arrived in Omaha, the NBU had had nearly a decade of drilling and study and team building.

(continued on page 140)

Response

The response at the NBU began weeks in advance of the arrival of the first patient. As the NBU was activated, the public information officer began to implement the communication strategy. This involved first notifying the staff and current patients of the hospital of the impending arrival of the EVD patient and activation of the NBU. The communication strategy included determining both internal and external messaging strategies, being as transparent as possible, and making sure that those inside the organization had relevant information before it was disseminated to the general public. Everyone involved was encouraged to ask questions. Then the public information officer worked with public health authorities and the media to keep the public informed and to minimize public fear associated with the patient's arrival. This included aggressive use of social media to help correct misperceptions, daily press conferences to update the press and the public, and working with patients and their families to keep the public updated on the patients' progress. The resulting culture of transparency helped reduce anxiety both inside and outside the organization.

Meanwhile, NBU staff readied the unit to receive the first patient and reviewed policies and procedures using just-in-time materials, videos, checklists, and other educational materials on subjects such as PPE use and staff temperature monitoring. The NBU activated its own Incident Command System as well as a dedicated incident command subsystem to oversee transport of the first patient from the airport to the unit. On arrival, the patient was transferred to a specially retrofitted ambulance staffed by emergency medical services (EMS) workers with special training in infection control and decontamination. The ambulance then transported the patient from the airport to the NBU, where NBU staff took over.

Between September 2014 and March 2015, the NBU treated three actual Ebola patients and monitored seven others who had been exposed but who turned out not to have contracted the disease. All but one of the patients survived, and there was no transmission of the virus to NBU staff.

Recovery and Moving Forward

The NBU has created a highly successful model for treating highly infectious patients, one that fosters interdisciplinary and vertical collaboration and results in significant esprit de corps on the part of the staff. Indeed, NBU staff experience little to no attrition, and there is a waiting list to join. However, no response is perfect, and NBU leaders continue to try to address identified shortcomings.

In debriefing and after-action reporting, staff identified a number of areas for improvement. Because NBU staff normally work in other areas of the hospital, it is critical to provide for the backfilling of those positions vacated by them during activation. Staff temperature monitoring was initially overwhelming, showing the need for further refinement of the procedures. Also, it was noted that no cost structures existed for the NBU response. While the incident command structure facilitated the procurement of necessary supplies and medications, the response was made more efficient by the development of cost structures for the activated unit.

Lessons learned through training and actual response at the NBU are being shared broadly at conferences and through the National Ebola Training and Education Center, a coalition comprising the University of Nebraska Medical Center, Emory University, and Bellevue Hospital Center in New York, in collaboration with the Centers for Disease Control and Prevention and the US Department of Health and Human Services' Office of the Assistant Secretary for Preparedness and Response. Together, these institutions and agencies are developing best practices for treatment and education, as well as creating a network of hospitals to help quickly identify, isolate, and treat patients with other highly infectious diseases besides Ebola. This is complex work that requires the cooperation of dozens of agencies and institutions and scores of people. (*See* Figure 9-3 to understand the complex nature of the relationships necessary for a successful emergency response.)

Standardized debriefing questionnaires that use a mix of closed-ended and open-ended questions can help give shape to the large amounts of data and opinion generated by the evaluation process. A simple way to gather feedback is to ask three open-ended questions: What went well? What needs improvement? Any other feedback? The staff person leading the after-action review could then ask questions related to the six critical areas. All involved parties should be encouraged or required to submit evaluations immediately following the exercise or response (*see* Figure 9-3 below for sample tools to use in this process).

Figure 9-3. **Planning for Patients with Infectious Disease**

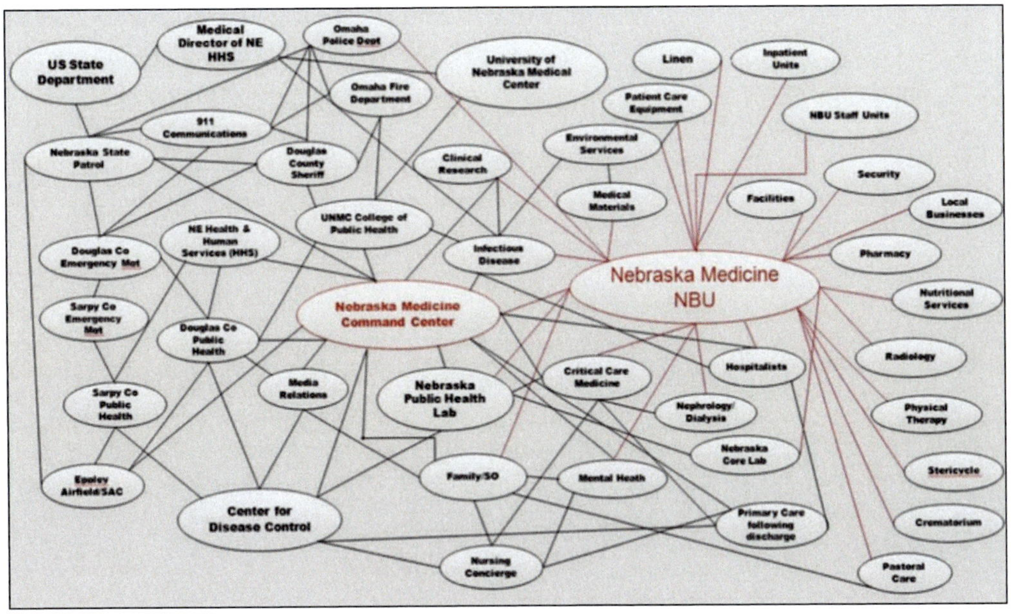

Figure 9-3 provides some of the key entities involved in planning for patients with infectious disease(s).

Source: University of Nebraska Medical Center/Nebraska Medicine. From Schwedhelm S, Lowe J, Boulter K. How to plan for the highly infectious disease patient. Presented at the Association of Healthcare Emergency Preparedness Professionals Annual Conference, Omaha, NE, Nov 18, 2015. Used with permission.

Organizations must evaluate the appropriateness of the response to the situation as well as the adequacy of that response. In other words, were the correct portions of the EOP initiated and did the resulting response allow the organization to manage the six critical areas of response over the required duration?

Observers and managers should consider the effectiveness of logistical planning, management of human resources, and staff training and education so that they can make informed recommendations as to improvements in preparedness, training, or the EOP. The availability and use of essential clinical and nonclinical supplies and equipment are also important elements of the evaluation. In addition, managers and planners need to evaluate the effectiveness of emergency policies, protocols, and procedures to ensure that they are having the desired effects and not creating confusion or hindering operations.

When the after-action report has been finalized, the emergency manager should evaluate the "big rock items" to determine where to focus finite energy and resources. Big rock items are those that, if not fixed, are highly likely to occur again. The smaller items should not be ignored but placed at a lower priority for follow-up. Deficiencies and opportunities for improvement in response, planning, and the EOP should be shared with department and unit managers and affected disciplines across the organization. Risk and emergency managers can aggregate data and synthesize observations to help create a broad picture for how to improve response. Comparing experiences with other organizations or between facilities can lead to an understanding of best practices. It may also be desirable to speak with representatives from vendors who supply critical emergency response technology, such as emergency power system monitoring, in order to get their input on how response can be improved.

Leadership Response

The deficiencies and opportunities for improvement identified in the evaluations are communicated to the improvement team responsible for monitoring environment of care and emergency management issues and to senior organization leadership. Senior leadership will establish priorities for performance improvement and determine which improvements in emergency preparedness will be implemented in the near term, and which will need to be tabled until sufficient resources or other strategic considerations are aligned to address more complex issues.

Modifying the EOP

As noted above, emergency planning should be a recursive process. Observations and recommendations for improvement should be reflected in modifications to the EOP, including, but not limited to, enhanced staff education and training, new mitigation activities, and changes to policies and procedures. The effectiveness of these modifications is then the subject of special scrutiny in the next exercise or response, and so on.

Figure 9-4. After-Action Review Sample

After-Action Review

Date of Event: Type of Disaster: Community ☐   Internal ☐   Other_____

Planned Event ☐

Actual Event ☐

Date reviewed by Emergency Management Committee or Manager:

Auditors	Areas or Activities Monitored

Type of Exercise: _____

Scenario: _____

Measurable Performance Expectations for the Six Critical Functions _____

1. Communications	Satisfactory ☐ Unsatisfactory ☐ NA ☐
Items to consider	**Comments from staff debriefing and auditors:**
√ Activation of emergency management all-hazards command structure	
√ Notification of appropriate members of peri-operative, surgical, and anesthesia services	
√ Communication with the media, suppliers, patient families	
√ Internal communications	
2. Resources and Assets	Satisfactory ☐ Unsatisfactory ☐ NA ☐
Items to consider	**Comments from staff debriefing and auditors:**
√ Additional resources located and addressed before receiving patients (stocking up)	
√ Plan for the replenishment of medical, nonmedical, and pharmaceuticals supplies	
√ Need for staff and staff family support addressed	
√ Stockpile inventories accessed	
3. Safety and Security	Satisfactory ☐ Unsatisfactory ☐ NA ☐
Items to consider	**Comments from staff debriefing and auditors:**
√ Internal and external security maintained	
√ Outside agencies identified in the facility during emergency operations	
√ Handling of hazardous materials	
√ Patients susceptible to "wandering" identified and monitored during emergencies	
√ Traffic external to the facility managed	

(continued on page 142)

Figure 9-4. **After-Action Review Sample** (continued)

4. Staff Responsibilities	Satisfactory ☐ Unsatisfactory ☐ NA ☐
Items to consider √ Staff awareness of their roles and responsibilities as defined in the influx or department-specific disaster policy √ Communication with licensed independent practitioners regarding their roles and to whom they report during emergency operations √ Methods to identify authorized personnel during the emergency	***Comments from staff debriefing and auditors:***
5. Utilities	Satisfactory ☐ Unsatisfactory ☐ NA ☐
Items to consider √ Alternate means of electricity, water for drinking and patient care, and water for equipment and sanitation √ Adequate fuel for building operations and transportation functions √ Alternate means for other essential utilities, e.g., ventilation, med gas/vacuum, elevators, etc.	***Comments from staff debriefing and auditors:***
6. Patient Clinical & Support Activities	Satisfactory ☐ Unsatisfactory ☐ NA ☐
Items to consider √ Scheduling, triage, assessment, treatment, admission, transfer, discharge, and evacuation. √ Needs of special populations e.g., pediatric, geriatric, and disabled √ Plans for personal hygiene and sanitation needs Plans for mortuary services √ Plans for documenting and tracking patient's clinical information	***Comments from staff debriefing and auditors:***

How was this event rated according to the Community Hazard Vulnerability Analysis (CHVA)?

Top Five Risk Occurrence/Response			
Risk Occurrence		**Risk Response**	
1	60%	1	67%
2	58%	2	63%
3	51%	3	61%
4	49%	4	60%
5	49%	5	58%

CHAPTER 9 | A Framework for Testing and Evaluation

Figure 9-4. **After-Action Review Sample** *(continued)*

CHVA Ratings					
Community Hazard Vulnerability Assessment Tool	**Probability**		**Human Impact**	**Property Impact**	**Business Impact**
	Likelihood of future occurrence and facility response		Percentage of population likely to be injured or killed under an average occurrence of the hazard	Percentage of properties likely to be affected under an average occurrence of the hazard	Percentage of businesses likely to be affected under an average occurrence of the hazard
	0 = N/A (implausible) 1 = Low (0–1 event / 30 years) 2 = Moderate (2–3 events / 30 years) 3 = High (4+ events / 30 years)		0 = N/A (no impact expected) 1 = Low (<1% affected) 2 = Moderate (1–10% affected) 3 = High (>10% affected)	0 = N/A (no impact expected) 1 = Low (<1% affected) 2 = Moderate (1–10% affected) 3 = High (>10% affected)	0 = N/A (no impact expected) 1 = Low (<1% affected) 2 = Moderate (1–10% affected) 3 = High (>10% affected)
	Occurrence	Response			
	3	1	1	1	2

Mitigation		Preparedness		Response		Recovery		Risk Occurrence	Risk Response
Internal (Jurisdictional)	External (Region/State)	Internal (Jurisdictional)	External (Region/State)	Internal (Jurisdictional)	External (Region/State)	Internal (Jurisdictional)	External (Region/State)	Relative threat (increases with percentage)	Relative threat (increases with percentage)
1 = Substantial 2 = Moderate 3 = Limited or none	1 = Substantial 2 = Moderate 3 = Limited or none	1 = Substantial 2 = Moderate 3 = Limited or none	1 = Substantial 2 = Moderate 3 = Limited or none	1 = Substantial 2 = Moderate 3 = Limited or none	1 = Substantial 2 = Moderate 3 = Limited or none	1 = Substantial 2 = Moderate 3 = Limited or none	1 = Substantial 2 = Moderate 3 = Limited or none	0%–100%	0%–100%
2	2	2	1	2	1	1	1	49%	16%

Does this event need to be added to the CHVA tool? ☐ Yes ☐ No
If yes, what should be added? (Insert here)

How was this event rated according to the 96 Hour Sustainability Grid?

Comparing this drill to past drills/events, what was noticeably improved or deficient?

What strengths were observed during the event?

What weaknesses were observed during the event?

Other comments:

(continued on page 144)

Figure 9-4. **After-Action Review Sample** (continued)

Follow-Up	Action Plan/Interim Measures	Person/Department Responsible	Anticipated Completion Date	Risk Rating 0–3
1.				
2.				
3.				

Interim measures required? Yes ☐ No ☐

Children's Hospital Colorado (CHCO) defines interim measures as urgent actions that must be resolved timely to reduce the imminent risk of irreparable harm to the facility and/or those individuals located in the facility. If interim measures are required, a risk rating of 3, these will be noted in the After-Action Review and on this form.

Notes relating to required interim measures:

_____
_____
_____
_____
_____
_____

Staff Debriefing		
Name	Title	Emergency Positions

Figure 9-4 provides after-action reports and other tools to evaluate an organization's emergency planning and response exercises.

Source: Niemer P. Children's Hospital Colorado. Aurora, CO. Used with permission.

IN SUMMARY

- Conduct annual evaluations of the hazard vulnerability analysis, objectives and scope of the EOP, and inventory to ensure that they are all current with evolving risks in the community, with capabilities of the organization, and with relationships with coalition partners.

- Design emergency exercises to test the organization's ability to handle complex or multiple emergencies. The exercises will also test critical areas of performance, including patient influx and evacuation.

- Hold a variety of drills and exercises designed to test both the stand-alone response capabilities of the organization and the effectiveness of its coordinated response with community partners. Tabletop exercises and computer simulations can be useful in some areas, but full-scale exercises and participation in communitywide exercises are necessary for thorough preparedness.

- Conduct thorough after-action debriefings and analyses to get a sense of where the organization is doing well and where it can improve its performance.

- Devise a Plan of Action that includes enhanced mitigation and preparedness activities, staff training required to address areas for improvement, and modifications to the EOP.

CHAPTER 10

After the Incident

> **STANDARDS FOCUS**
>
> **EM.02.01.01** The organization has an Emergency Operations Plan.
>
> **IM.01.01.03** The organization plans for continuity of its information management processes.

> **AT A GLANCE**
> - Restoring to normal operations
> - Continuity of operations
> - Downtime and recovery
> - Ceasing services

Why Is This Critical?

Emergencies push organizations to their very limits and sometimes beyond. Facilities may be damaged, supplies may be depleted, and recordkeeping may fall behind. The ability of the organization to operate at normal levels could be compromised, and its buildings may not be immediately usable. The organization's priority, after emergency operations are terminated, should be to get its facilities back up and running normally as soon as possible. How quickly recovery can happen depends on many factors, and in the worst cases recovery may require services or structures to be offline for months. The resilience of health care organizations, which relies on good planning and preparation, contributes to the resilience of the communities they serve.

> **WHO IS INVOLVED?**
> - Organization leadership
> - Facilities managers
> - Clinical engineers
> - Vendors and suppliers
> - Insurance companies
> - Administrative leadership
> - Safety officers
> - Emergency managers
> - Finance
> - Department managers

Key Concepts for Recovery

Recovering from the effects of an emergency is not an immediate process. Health care organizations and the communities in which they are located need time to transition from the heightened operations of an emergency situation to the usual operations of regular patient care. The attention given to the first three phases should not diminish during recovery. Additional resources over and beyond those given in the response phase may be necessary. The scope and duration of downtime may also require the need to utilize Incident Command or project management philosophies for effective management or oversight. An organization's successful recovery from an emergency relies on the resiliency of relationships developed in the Emergency Operations Plan (EOP). Organizations identify their needs and partner with community agencies, vendors, health care systems, and others to provide safe and timely services to patients while they implement plans to return to normal operations as soon as possible.

Restoring Normal Operations

Restoring the organization's facilities to normal operation as quickly as possible is the final phase of emergency management. An organization's degree of preparedness and response

149

determines how quickly it can recover from an emergency. The EOP, when combined with a comprehensive continuity of operations (COOP) plan, should provide a robust framework for recovery from emergencies. The emergency management team can best prepare by building a recovery plan that is adaptable to a wide range of emergency circumstances. Because the organization may not be in a position to fulfill its core mission in the wake of a disaster, having a COOP plan in place is important. Managers should plan in advance how to integrate COOP principals into the four phases of emergency management: mitigation, preparedness, response, and recovery.

Continuity of Operations

There are a variety of competing programs related to COOP, including, but not limited to, information technology disaster recovery (IT DR), business continuity planning (BCP), and continuity of government. What is similar in all of these programs, including COOP, is that they are focused on maintaining essential functions, disaster recovery, and recovery operations. Organizations need to understand how their facilities operate to build effective plans to maintain operations during downtime. COOP is the process by which health care organizations can build these plans. The concept behind COOP is to ensure that the facilities' essential functions (core mission of a department or area) are maintained.

Why is COOP important to health care? The simple answer is to ensure continuity of care. If your facility can no longer maintain its essential functions, the likelihood of department/facility closure or evacuation will significantly increase. Other reasons COOP is important include the following:
- Competitive advantage
- Operational efficiency
- Sustainability—succession planning
- Risk identification and reduction
- Leadership engagement

To assist emergency managers and other health care leaders understand the value of collecting data and building a comprehensive COOP plan, let's review the following scenario. A large multidisciplinary ambulatory clinic closed operations due to a public health concern. It is anticipated that the building will be closed for at least two weeks with limited staff access. All patients, visitors, and staff have been evacuated.

Is this a likely scenario for your facility? How would your facility handle its response? COOP planning assists the incident command team by having immediate access to relevant data in a timely manner. Prior to building an effective COOP plan, command staff would have to meet with individual leaders to determine their plans for the downtime. This entails a significant number of questions to obtain pertinent information. With an effective COOP plan, the data have already been collected and verified and may already be utilized in decision making. Which way do you think is more effective: waiting to collect the data—or having access to the data immediately?

There are many components to an effective COOP plan, and it is up to the facility to determine how to implement it and which components to integrate. To assist emergency managers, Children's Hospital Colorado* (CHCO), a private, not-for-profit pediatric Level 1 trauma center in a seven-state region seeing patients from Montana through New Mexico, has created a health care–specific COOP tool entitled Operational Profile Template—Continuity of Operations (COOP), which is designed to assist with COOP plan development and implementation. The tool is available on the CHCO website at http://www.childrenscolorado.org/health-professionals/clinical-resources/emergency-management/.

Essential Functions

Recovery can be an uneven process. Some essential functions may need to be restored more quickly than others. The Federal Emergency Management Agency (FEMA) defines essential functions as the critical activities that are performed by an organization, particularly after a disruption of normal activities. CHCO defines essential functions as the fundamental roles that a department fulfills within the context of facility operations. No matter the definition used, the basic concept of essential functions is to determine which function(s) need to be restored first.

Developing essential functions will take time, as it is easy to confuse functions with processes. Think of the department as the title of a book. The chapters are the functions, and the processes are the pages that fill the chapters. For example, the essential function(s) (chapters) of the emergency department are triage, assessment, and stabilization. All of the numerous processes that take place within an emergency department to perform these essential function(s) fall under the chapters of triage, assessment, and stabilization. It is possible for a department to have multiple essential functions.

COOP Versus the EOP

COOP is the initiative that ensures that all departments are able to *continue operation* of their essential functions under a broad range of circumstances. The EOP *describes how* a facility will respond to and recover from an event. Integration of COOP and the EOP can be an overwhelming prospect for emergency managers, as both programs require extensive knowledge of health care culture and facility/community preparedness and response. The relationship between COOP and the EOP is symbiotic. While one can survive without the other, combining them creates a stronger system from which the EOP acts as an extension of COOP. COOP is the root system from which the EOP thrives.

Similarities with the EOP
- All-hazards approach
- Follows the four phases of emergency management
- Risk identification and reduction—hazard vulnerability analyses
- Senior leadership support

Differences from the EOP
- Broad operational focus
- Emphasis on redundancy
- Identification of/prioritization based on essential functions

Building a bridge between COOP and the EOP requires analysis and operational integration for the programs to remain consistent and functional. Emergency managers need to assess a variety of risk factors that influence health care operations and accommodate an all-hazards approach for risk minimization. The hazard vulnerability analysis (HVA), when conducted properly, will assist the emergency manager in identifying and focusing limited resources. HVAs should assess risks that have the highest likelihood of impacting operations. A common mistake among emergency managers is to limit the type and number of HVA risks. A robust HVA should identify blind spots and help target limited resources. The community or coalition HVA is another risk assessment that should be included as long as the events are consistently defined and rated among the participating partners.

Plan Activation

The first question often asked about COOP is when the plan should be activated. The entire COOP plan, or elements thereof, may be activated whenever an event disrupts or threatens to disrupt normal business operations for an extended period of time. If the information in the business impact analysis is useful during response and recovery phases, it should be used.

Downtime and Recovery

What is downtime? A common misconception of downtime is that it is limited to an information technology failure, such as the loss of electronic medical records. CHCO defines downtime as the period of time when something, such as a building system failure, aspect, or process that contributes to the essential function, is not in operation. In other words, anything that disrupts normal operations is downtime. Do you have downtime and recovery procedures in place for anything that shuts down your operations (IT, facilities, staffing, equipment failure, and so on)?

Similar to the EOP, downtime and recovery procedures should be written as a framework for each type of downtime and then integrated at the department level. Figure 10-1 on page 153 shows a sample form that could be used at the department level to help document downtime and recovery procedures.

Capacity Builder

Implementing the COOP Plan

The following steps may be used in the development of a COOP plan. Individual facilities should add or remove steps based on their needs[1]:

1. Create a steering committee comprised of a diverse team of leaders who understand operations, business continuity, and risk.
2. Develop a COOP plan and implementation strategy.
3. Develop a business impact analysis interview tool.
4. Conduct manager interviews.
5. Interview departments where data can be collected, and develop reports based on available data.
6. Integrate the business impact analysis and data into a relational database.
7. Test/modify the COOP plan.
8. Reevaluate the COOP plan and integrate with other systems.

REFERENCE

1. Niemer P, Cantrell N. Operational Profile Template—Continuity of Operations (COOP). Aurora, CO: Children's Hospital of Colorado, 2015. Accessed Jun 26, 2016. https://www.childrenscolorado.org/health-professionals/clinical-resources/emergency-management/.

Figure 10-1. Downtime and Recovery Documentation Form

Downtime Procedures			
System Failure Example	Downtime Procedures	Recovery Procedures	Failure Point (0 Minutes–90 Days)
IT Application [A]			
IT Application [A]			
Electrical—Generator(s) work			
Electrical—No generator(s)			
Flood			
Natural gas			
Telephones			
Water (potable)			
Water leak			
Water (nonpotable)			
Temperature monitoring			
Fire alarm/Fire sprinkler			
Natural gas leak			
Sewer stoppage			
Ventilation systems (HVAC)			
Staffing			
Supplies			
Medical equipment			

IT, information technology; HVAC, heating, ventilating, and air-conditioning.

Figure 10-1 can be used as a template for department managers to document periods when normal operations are disrupted and capture the recovery procedures followed. The first column would be filled in as various system failures occur—the items shown in this template are for example only.

Source: Niemer P. Children's Hospital Colorado. Aurora, CO. Used with permission.

To help develop comprehensive downtime and recovery procedures, CHCO identified, modified, and created five work groups. The five work groups consist of downtime communications, forms, utilities, policy/procedures, and IT DR. The goal of each work group is to cast a wide enough net to cover any and all aspects of emergency management processes related to COOP and downtime and recovery. While the scope is quite large, it helps break down the barriers between individual departments. Organizations should evaluate their existing downtime and recovery processes to determine if work groups should be developed.

Recovery Activities

Health care organizations are a critical resource to the communities they serve and the people they employ. An organization's ability to maintain the quality and continuity of care in the face and aftermath of an emergency is of utmost importance. Their continued operation depends on several critical functions described in the following sections.

After-Action Review

The recovery phase should be a time when organization leadership considers the possibilities for improvements, upgrades, and mitigation for the future. Catastrophic damage, while disruptive, presents an opportunity to "build it back better." The after-action review (AAR) process is an important tool for documenting feedback and next steps. The six critical areas of communications, resources and assets, safety and security, staff responsibilities, utilities, and patient clinical and support activities should be reviewed. Some organizations also evaluate infection prevention and IT, as both areas have a high likelihood of being involved. (*See* Chapter 9 for more information on testing and evaluation.)

Finances

Does the organization have sufficient funding to support recovery operations and near-term improvement projects? Organization leaders need to maintain business plans that include financial recovery. Such a plan will incorporate existing funds with claims paid by insurance and any other recovery and restoration funds that the organization can obtain, such as disaster assistance grants from FEMA. A solid understanding of the organization's current financial position is essential to planning every part of the recovery phase. The Centers for Disease Control and Prevention (CDC) has created a hospital disaster preparedness budget model, which is a Microsoft Excel template designed to assist health care executives in making the kinds of plans and budget decisions that can help identify, monitor, and manage the funds required for recovery efforts. The tool is available on the CDC website at http://www.cdc.gov/phpr/healthcare/hospitals.htm.

Capacity Builder

The Centers for Medicare and Medicaid Services (CMS) provides a template and instructions for completing an after-action report and improvement plan: https://www.cms.gov/Medicare/Provider-Enrollment-and-Certification/SurveyCertEmergPrep/Templates-Checklists.html.

The Illinois Emergency Management Agency (IEMA) is one of many other organizations that provides numerous templates and resources to plan and evaluate exercises: http://www.illinois.gov/iema/Training/Pages/HSEEP.aspx.

CHAPTER 10 | After the Incident

Case in Point
Cape Canaveral Hospital Hit with Three Hurricanes in Seven Weeks

Health First–Cape Canaveral Hospital is a 150-bed hospital located in Cocoa Beach, Florida. It is part of the Health First network, a not-for-profit health care network made up of four hospitals and an array of wellness centers and other facilities, serving east central Florida. Cape Canaveral is home to a birthing center and a 21-bed Level 2 emergency department. In the summer of 2004 Cape Canaveral Hospital was struck by three powerful hurricanes, which forced two evacuations.

Preparation

Being on the Atlantic coast of Florida, emergency planners for Health First put a high priority on hurricane planning and evacuation planning. They created an array of cross-disciplinary teams to consider issues, including child and elder care, coordination with outside entities such as law enforcement and fire departments, the creation of a special needs shelter, evacuation procedures, Joint Commission compliance, census management, poststorm damage assessment, and so on. One team is tasked each year with updating a pamphlet called the Hurricane Preparedness Guidebook, which is given to staff and included in the new-hires packet. Evacuation drills are held each May to prepare for the onset of hurricane season, and Health First has developed a Web-based tool to help organize and track the progress of evacuations.

Because information is critical to decision making, particularly when it comes to evacuation decisions in an evolving weather emergency, Health First employs a variety of communications equipment, including a satellite phone in the command center, Internet, ham radio, UHF and VHF radios, and televisions with both cable and satellite feeds. These tools allow emergency managers and staff to stay abreast of storm developments and communicate with one another as the situation evolves.

In addition, standing agreements govern the delivery of fuel and supplies and on-site support from local law enforcement.

Incident and Response

The first of the three hurricanes, Charley, arrived on August 13, 2004. A west-to-east hurricane, the storm made landfall on the other side of the peninsula, which likely softened the impact on Cape Canaveral Hospital. However, the storm was still sufficiently powerful to cause a six-hour power loss. Three weeks later, on September 2, the hospital was hit by a second hurricane, Frances, which dropped more than 20 inches of rain on Cocoa Beach and did nearly $9 billion in property damage. Cape Canaveral Hospital fell within the mandatory evacuation area. Of the 72 patients in the hospital at the time, 35 were able to be discharged, and hospital staff managed to evacuate the other 37 within six hours. The hospital was struck a third time, by hurricane Jeanne, on September 25, which caused a further $6.9 billion in property damage. Again, the hospital fell under a mandatory evacuation order, and the staff were forced to evacuate and transfer 56 patients, which they did in four hours.

(continued on page 156)

Aftermath and Recovery

Obviously, the recovery from such an extreme series of weather events was long and difficult. There was extensive damage to the hospital itself, including water intrusion. Patients had to be relocated to other hospitals in the network and beyond. Disaster Medical Assistance Teams (DMATs) were brought in to deal with an influx of patients that coincided with the hospital's attempts to lower its census. One of the chief challenges in the aftermath of the storms was providing shelter and child care to hospital staff, including many whose homes were destroyed or heavily damaged. Indeed, following Hurricane Jeanne, more than two hundred of the hospital's associates were seeking assistance with storm-related damage. Health First utilized space at its other facilities, including a hospice facility, to house displaced staff and provide child care, so that the staff could continue to work. They also provided cash advances to help employees deal with short-term needs as the community rebounded.

In response to this experience, Health First and Cape Canaveral Hospital made a number of changes in policy and procedures. These included the addition of a satellite television feed to the command center to serve as a backup to the cable. It was decided to send a representative from the hospital to the local emergency operations center any time there was the potential for an emergency management event. This includes hurricanes and other storms as well as launches at the nearby Kennedy Space Center. They continue to refine their Web-based evacuation tracking tool and their evacuation procedures as they plan for the next hurricane, which they know is coming.

Facilities and Equipment

Damage to facilities and infrastructure may necessitate a prolonged shutdown of operations. Repair and replacement of equipment and systems can stretch into weeks and months, and sometimes years, because many components may have to be custom made to fulfill the needs of the facility and the requirements of Joint Commission standards and laws and regulations. Organizations need to have a plan for what to do if the organization is unable to provide care and services for an extended period of time. This includes working with state and local authorities, insurance providers, FEMA, and other agencies.

Many different kinds of emergencies can cause damage to facilities. From fires to floods to earthquakes and bombs, a full damage assessment must be among the organization's first priorities after the emergency has subsided. Structural and electrical engineers, as well as building and clinical engineers, will need to assess the safety of the buildings and the condition of critical systems, including the utilities systems; heating, ventilating, and air-conditioning (HVAC); fire suppression; information management; and other systems. Facility assessments are critical information streams that will be used by the incident command team to determine operational priorities. Facilities-related risk assessments should be reviewed and updated annually and after each event.

Alternative Care Locations

Even if buildings are safe to use, emergency planners must consider whether or not the organization can support the full range of patient care, treatment, and services. If not, they will need to plan in advance for some services to be provided through coalition partnerships, performed at other facilities operated by the parent organization, contracted out, or temporarily suspended. For example, the plan may include a protocol for arranging the provision of any services that may need to be contracted out, such as laundry or lab services, while the organization is recovering. Having a standing list of alternative care locations and possible providers of such services saves time, and having preexisting agreements and working relationships with principals at those entities can facilitate smoother transitions for patients. Some less critical services or operations may be suspended for a longer period of time or relocated to another facility.

Chief among the organization's concerns should be the disposition of patients. If the facility is no longer capable of supporting their care, patients will need to be relocated to other facilities. The organization will cease receiving new patients and will work through the local emergency operations center and health care coalition partners to transfer any remaining patients to the care of other organizations based on patient type (medical, surgical, chronic, behavioral health) and acuity. Clinical records, medications, supplies, and equipment supporting the transfer of these patients will be provided to the extent possible, and staff will travel with patients or be placed in other facilities to the extent possible. Plans for transportation of patients and records should be in place beforehand to expedite the process. The COOP plan should incorporate all aspects of alternative care locations, both primary and secondary.

Staffing

It must be determined as quickly as possible whether the organization has sufficient staff to resume normal operations. Staff may be injured or ill, or just overwhelmed with personal or family issues and in need of time to recover. Provisions should be made to give staff breaks and extra downtime in a way that does not leave the organization understaffed. In addition, staff may need extra services such as child care, pet care, elder care, and financial, counseling, or mental health services. For communitywide disasters, some organizations, as part of their emergency planning, obtain supplies of cash with which to make loans to staff in the event that ATMs are offline and banks are closed. (These loans are repaid via deductions over time from their paychecks.) In some cases, organizations will facilitate the hiring of contractors to begin repairs to the homes of staff to help alleviate anxiety. Helping connect staff with providers of these sorts of services can speed their return to work in the wake of an emergency.

It is not optimal to determine staff strategies during an event. A comprehensive list of staffing strategies should be developed as part of the COOP plan/EOP. (*See* Chapter 6 on preparing staff to respond.)

Sample staffing strategies may include, but are not limited to, the following:
- 12 hours on, 12 hours off
- Re-allocate existing staff
- Labor pool
- Overtime
- Contract staff
- Leadership backfill
- Memoranda of understanding or other agreements
- Volunteers
- Retired practitioners
- Retired staff
- Close/restrict nonessential functions
- Suspend vacations and paid time off
- Utilize staff from other partner facilities
- Extend shift change
- Cancel educational events/conferences

Case in Point
Bon Secours Baltimore: Better than Before

Certain internal or external disasters provide the opportunity to improve services to patients and surrounding communities. Bon Secours Baltimore Health System is a full-service health system in Baltimore. At its core is a 72-bed acute care hospital, which provides primary and emergency care and a vast array of community outreach services. In the aftermath of civil unrest in 2015 that resulted in thefts, vandalism, and disruption of staff and patient access to the hospital, Bon Secours took specific steps to improve future resilience in relation to key lessons learned:

- Practice lockdown procedures.
- Review security of treatment program buildings.
- Develop civil unrest guide.
- Identify separate areas for victims and police.
- Provide emotional impact.
- Define vendor expectations.
- Identify map of area with hospital assets.
- Plan for incident commander relief during extended events.

Because Bon Secours has a core mission of community support, the full recovery and resilience of the health system was entwined with the recovery of the community. To enhance already robust community outreach programs, Bon Secours initiated planning for extended services to at-risk youths ages 14 to 24, recognizing the opportunity to expand the health care workforce in ways that benefitted both the hospital and the community:

- Youth summer employment
- Job readiness and leadership training
- Nurturing parent skills-building workshops
- Reentry program for young offenders
- Career exploration pilot project
- Reading partners
- GED prep courses

Like Bon Secours, several other hospitals in Baltimore recognized the importance of identifying community assets and enhancing collaborative partnerships in response to this state of emergency; they included in their recovery efforts plans and funding to improve the continuity of the medical and social service network throughout the at-risk neighborhoods.

Ceasing Services

A recovery phase may be very short term, such as reorganizing the emergency department following the treatment of 12 car accident victims, or significantly longer and more complex, as in the case of a hospital that sustains earthquake damage, loses all electrical power, and therefore has to evacuate. If the organization ceases services temporarily or permanently, it will affect its accreditation status.

Notifying The Joint Commission

The organization should inform The Joint Commission immediately if a prolonged shutdown is necessary, by contacting the organization's assigned account executive or calling The Joint Commission. It should work with The Joint Commission to develop a plan and a timeline for recovery and resumption of services. Joint Commission expertise can be invaluable in developing these plans and expediting the process. Local, state, and federal authorities should also be informed of the shutdown and kept apprised of recovery plans and timelines so that community health care needs do not go unmet while the organization is recovering.

Impact of Cessation of Services on Accreditation Status

When The Joint Commission is informed of a cessation of services, it will work with organization leadership to address the impact of the cessation on accreditation status and ensure that when the facility resumes operations the safety and quality of care are of a sufficiently high level. The Joint Commission sets out four categories of cessation, each with its own impact on accreditation status:

1. **Cessation of up to 30 days:** For organizations that resume services within 30 days, there will be no change in their Joint Commission accreditation status. In most cases The Joint Commission will not conduct a survey upon resumption of services, and the clock on any outstanding compliance issues will pause during the cessation.
2. **Cessation of up to 90 days:** Organizations that resume operations between 31 and 90 days after a disaster will be subject to an extension survey, the length and scope of which will be determined by the circumstances surrounding the cessation.
3. **Cessation of up to six months:** Organizations that resume services from 91 days to six months after a disaster will be subject to two on-site surveys. The first will take place one to two weeks following the resumption of services to assess the environment of care. The second will take place four months following resumption of services and will focus on sustained compliance.
4. **Cessation of more than six months:** Organizations that cease services for more than six months will lose their accreditations status. If they resume services, they will have to reapply for accreditation. During the cessation The Joint Commission will work with the health care organization and relevant government agencies to help the organization resume operations and regain its accreditation status.

> **IN SUMMARY**
> - Restore normal operations as quickly as possible, including making repairs to facilities, financial recovery, insurance, clinical records, and ongoing patient tracking.
> - Develop a written COOP plan and include business impact analysis documents for each department.
> - Develop downtime and recovery procedures to assist during an event.
> - Begin to rotate staff off the line to give them time off following the emergency.
> - Identify primary and secondary alternative care locations in the event that services need to be relocated.
> - In case of protracted recovery, contact community partners and authorities to help ensure the availability of health care in the community.
> - In the event that the facility must be shut down for a long period, work with The Joint Commission and other partners to expedite recovery.

Glossary

active shooter An individual actively engaged in killing or attempting to kill people in a confined and populated area; in most cases, active shooters use firearms, and there's no pattern or method to their selection of victims.

active threat A situation that occurs without warning, quickly degenerates, and has the potential to cause death or serious injury.

after-action report An analysis of an emergency response to an event or exercise that evaluates strengths and weaknesses of the response and identifies areas that need improvement.

"all-hazards" approach An emergency management methodology that supports a general response capability that is sufficiently nimble to address a range of emergencies of different duration, scale, and cause.

alternative care site A location operated by businesses and agencies other than the health care organization where lower-acuity patients may be transferred for continued care and treatment during an emergency.

annually One year from the date of the last event, plus or minus 30 days. Synonymous with every 12 months, once a year, or every year.

best practice A clinical, scientific, or professional practice that is recognized by a majority of professionals in a particular field as being exemplary. These practices are typically evidence based and consensus driven.

cessation Temporary or permanent conclusion of services.

competence The knowledge, skills, ability, and behavior that a person possesses to perform tasks correctly and skillfully.

continuity of operations The ability to continue services or essential functions under a range of circumstances.

credentialing The process of obtaining, verifying, and assessing the qualifications of a practitioner to provide care or services in or for a health care organization.

crisis standards of care Standards that represent a substantial change in usual health care operations and the level of care it is possible to deliver, which is made necessary by a pervasive (for example, pandemic influenza) or catastrophic (for example, earthquake, hurricane) disaster.

debriefing The process of questioning a process or undertaking.

decontamination Removing or neutralizing dangerous materials and/or substances.

disaster A type of emergency that, due to its complexity, scope, or duration, threatens an organization's capabilities and requires outside assistance to sustain care, safety, or security functions.

disaster volunteers People who willingly offer assistance to overwhelmed health care organizations and community agencies to help provide care for disaster victims.

drills Emergency exercises designed to test individual facets of an organization's response capabilities so that emergency planners can evaluate individual parts of the Emergency Operations Plan.

---

emergency An unexpected or sudden event that significantly disrupts an organization's ability to provide care, treatment, or services or that results in a sudden, significantly changed or increased demand for those services. Emergencies can be either human-made or natural (such as an electrical system failure or a tornado), or a combination of both, and they exist on a continuum of severity.

emergency health care coalitions A collaborative network of health care organizations and their respective public- and private-sector response partners that serve as a multiagency coordinating group to assist with mitigation, preparedness, response, and recovery activities related to health care organization disaster operations.

emergency management The overarching discipline that ensures that organizations are building and testing plans utilizing the four phases of emergency management: mitigation, preparedness, response, and recovery.

Emergency Management Plan (EMP) *See* Emergency Operations Plan (EOP).

emergency manager Individual responsible for overseeing and facilitating emergency preparedness activities.

Emergency Operations Plan (EOP) An organization's written document that describes the process it would implement for managing emergencies or disasters that could disrupt the organization's ability to provide care, treatment, and services. The six critical areas of response in the EOP are communications, assets and resources, safety and security, staff responsibilities, utilities, and patient clinical and support activities. Called an Emergency Management Plan (EMP) in ambulatory and behavioral health care settings.

electronic medical record (EMR) An electronic version of a patient's medical record.

evacuation Removing individuals from a dangerous situation. An evacuation could be partial (at the site of an incident, affect certain groups of patients or areas within the facility, horizontally move individuals beyond corridor fire doors and/or smoke zones on the same floor, vertically move individuals from one floor[s] to the floor[s] above or below) or be complete and encompass the entire organization.

exercise An activity conducted by an organization to practice, train, and/or drill for emergency events using mock scenarios intended to gauge the effectiveness of the organization's Emergency Operations Plan. See also functional exercise; tabletop exercise.

---

first responders Individuals certified to provide medical care in emergencies before more highly trained medical personnel arrive on the scene.

functional exercise An exercise that validates the coordination of the emergency response activities within the organization, including collaboration with planning and response partners. It is an operations-based exercise that is action-oriented and designed to validate plans, policies, agreements, and procedures; clarify roles and responsibilities; and identify resource gaps in an operational environment.

---

hazard vulnerability analysis (HVA) A process for identifying potential emergencies and the direct and indirect effects these emergencies may have on an organization's operations and the demand for its services.

Hospital Incident Command System (HICS) A formal management system that enables health care organizations to remain operational during an emergency and promotes the restoration of services after the emergency has been managed. HICS defines roles related to the command staff, operations, planning, logistics, and finance/operations.

---

incident commander An individual responsible for all aspects of an emergency response, including developing incident objectives and priorities and managing and monitoring all incident operations.

Incident Command Structure (ICS)—The combination of personnel, procedures, communications, equipment, and facilities operating within a common organizational structure, designed to aid in managing an emergency of any size and scope.

influx *See* surge event.

inventory, 96-hour The health care organization's ability to provide communications, resources and assets, security and safety, staff, utilities, or patient care to sustain operations for at least 96 hours.

---

leader An individual who sets expectations, develops plans, and implements procedures to assess and improve the quality of the organization's governance, management, and clinical and support functions and processes. At a minimum, leaders include members of the governing body and medical staff, the chief executive officer and other senior managers, the nurse executive, clinical leaders, and staff members in leadership positions within the organization.

licensed independent practitioner An individual permitted by law and by the organization to provide care, treatment, and services without direction or supervision. A licensed independent practitioner operates within the scope of his or her license, consistent with individually granted clinical privileges.

---

meal, ready to eat (MRE) A contained, long-lasting meal designed and packaged to withstand rough conditions. MREs have a shelf life of several years.

medical equipment Fixed and portable equipment used for the diagnosis, treatment, monitoring, and direct care of individuals.

medical supplies Medical items, usually of a disposable nature, such as bandages, sterile drapes, and suture materials. These supplies differ from permanent or durable items, such as medical equipment and devices.

mitigation Actions taken in attempting to reduce the probability, severity, and/or impact of a potential emergency; first of the four phases of emergency management.

National Incident Management System (NIMS) A nationwide framework created by the US government that provides an all-hazards approach to emergency management and coordinates the responsibilities of organizations and jurisdictions.

---

operations The activities involved in running a health care organization.

outbreak The occurrence of more than the expected number of cases of disease, injury, or other health conditions among a specific group during a specified time frame.

---

patient An individual who receives care, treatment, or services. Synonyms used by various health care fields include resident, patient and family unit, individual served, consumer, health care consumer, customer, and beneficiary.

personal protective equipment (PPE) Clothing and other equipment worn to minimize exposure to serious workplace injuries and illnesses that may result from contact with chemical, radiological, physical, electrical, mechanical, or other workplace hazards. PPE may include gloves, safety glasses, shoes, earplugs or muffs, hard hats, respirators, coveralls, vests, and full body suits.

preparedness Actions taken to build capacity and identify resources that may be used if an emergency occurs; second of the four phases of emergency management.

privileging The process whereby the specific scope and content of patient care services (that is, clinical privileges) are authorized for a health care practitioner by a health care organization based on evaluation of the individual's credentials and performance.

public information officer (PIO) The designated spokesperson that coordinates with the crisis communications team.

receiving facility A health care organization to which a patient is transferred.

recovery Strategies, actions, and individual responsibilities taken to restore services after an emergency; last of the four phases of emergency management.

response Actions taken and procedures implemented when an emergency occurs; third of the four phases of emergency management.

safety The degree to which an intervention in the health care environment is free of risk for a patient and other persons, including workers. Safety risks may arise from the performance of tasks, from the structure of the physical environment, or from situations beyond the organization's control (such as weather).

security Protection of people and property against harm or loss (for example, workplace violence, theft, access to medications). Security incidents may be caused by persons from outside or inside the organization.

shelter A nontreatment setting that provides emergency housing and, where needed, protection for individuals.

stockpile A storage of essential supplies such as medicines and food rations in anticipation of a future shortage.

surge event An unexpected influx of patients that has the potential to or has overwhelmed organizational resources (for example, mass casualty, epidemic, flu).

tabletop exercise An exercise that involves key personnel discussing simulated scenarios and is used to assess plans, policies, and procedures. It is a discussion-based exercise that familiarizes participants with current plans, policies, agreements, and procedures, or may also be used to develop new plans, policies, agreements, and procedures.

triage Sorting and allocating treatment of patients during and after an emergency or disaster according to severity of condition to maximize the number of survivors.

utility systems Building systems that support the use and function of the physical environment, such as heating, cooling, water distribution, and vertical transport systems.

volunteer practitioner An individual who is not a licensed independent practitioner but who is required by law and regulation to have a license, certification, or registration to volunteer his or her services during a disaster.

vulnerable population A group of individuals who may have particular needs that set them apart from a more general patient population in their ability to anticipate, cope with, resist, and recover from the impacts of disasters. These populations may include children and adolescents, mental health patients, and the elderly.

Index

A

Accreditation status and cessation of services, 105, 160
Active shooter incidents
    access control during, 67, 69
    case study, Health First–Palm Bay Hospital incident, 67
    guide for procedures to follow during, 67
    mitigation activities to reduce vulnerability to, 15
    possible hazards related to, 2
    preparedness and response plans for, vii, viii, xii, 8, 69
    run, hide, or fight response, 69, 88
    staff training for, 69, 88
After-action debriefings, 137, 143–146, 147
Alternative care sites, 17, 22, 34, 52, 62, 115, 127, 156–157, 160
Ambulatory health care organizations
    Emergency Management (EM) standards for, xiii
    Emergency Management Plan requirement for, xv
American Academy of Pediatrics (AAP), 118
American Association for Respiratory Care (AARC), 58–59
Assets. *See* Resources and assets
Assistant Secretary for Preparedness and Response (ASPR), 7, 87, 90, 141

B

Baltimore
    Bon Secours Baltimore Health System recovery and resilience case study, 158
    coordination between community partners and health care organizations during civil unrest in, 18
    University of Maryland Medical Center continuity of operations during civil unrest and riots case study, 70–71
    University of Maryland Medical Center snow storm event case study, 19–20

Bathing, 101
Behavior, disruptive, 66
Behavioral health care organizations
    Emergency Management (EM) standards for, xiii
    emergency management for patients in, 62
    Emergency Management Plan requirement for, xv
Belgium, terrorist attack in, 72
Bellevue Hospital Center, 141
Beth Israel Deaconess Medical Center, Boston, xi
Beth Israel Deaconess Medical Center communitywide exercise and operating room evacuation drill case study, 134–136
Big rock items, 142
Biological events. *See* Chemical, biological, radiological, nuclear, explosive (CBRNE) events
Boil water notices, 100–101, 102–103
Bomb threat drills, 73
Bon Secours Baltimore Health System recovery and resilience case study, 158
Boston Marathon bombing, 72
Budget and financial plan development, 56, 154
Building collapses, 1, 2
Business continuity planning (BCP), 47, 150

C

Cape Canaveral Hospital hurricane events and and recovery case study, 155–156
Carilion Franklin Memorial Hospital staff training case study, 82–83
Case studies
    Beth Israel Deaconess Medical Center communitywide exercise and operating room evacuation drill, 134–136
    Bon Secours Baltimore Health System recovery and resilience, 158

Cape Canaveral Hospital hurricane events and recovery, 155–156
Carilion Franklin Memorial Hospital staff training, 82–83
Crozer-Keystone Health System security measures surrounding Pope's visit, 14–15
Health First–Palm Bay Hospital active shooter incident, 67
Highland Clarksburg Hospital snow storm event, 19–20
Kona Community Hospital earthquake response, 126–127
Mercy Hospital Joplin tornado event and evacuation, 92–93
Sutter Medical Center backup power failure, 108–109
University of Maryland Medical Center continuity of operations during civil unrest and riots, 70–71
University of Maryland Medical Center snow storm event, 19–20
University of Nebraska Medical Center/Nebraska Biocontainment Unit Ebola patients treatment, 9, 39, 139–141
Yale New Haven Health IT outage, 47–49
Centers for Disease Control and Prevention (CDC)
    Chemical Hazards Emergency Medical Management (CHEMM) program and CHEMPACKs, 57
    communication with, 44
    Ebola treatment and best practices development, 141
    hospital disaster preparedness budget model, 154
    staff training on safety protection policies, 88
    Strategic National Stockpile (SNS), 57, 58–59
    ventilators from SNS, 58–59
Centers for Medicare & Medicaid Services (CMS)
    after-action review template, 154
    emergency preparedness information, 7
    final rule, xv
    regulation and policy updates, 7
Cessation of services, 105, 159, 160
Chemical, biological, radiological, nuclear, explosive (CBRNE) events. *See also* Decontamination and decontamination facilities
    EOP, safety and security threats, and prevention of, 68
    isolation plans and procedures, 76–77
    medications for, obtaining and replenishing supply of, 57
    personnel safety in laboratories, 68
    possible hazards related to, 2
    staff training for response to, 88
    staff training on control/isolation precautions, 90
    state agencies for response to, 76
    triage location for patients, 113
Chemical Hazards Emergency Medical Management (CHEMM) program and CHEMPACKS, 57

Children's Hospital Colorado (CHCO), 150–154
Civil unrest incidents
    case studies
        Bon Secours Baltimore Health System recovery and resilience, 158
        University of Maryland Medical Center continuity of operations during, 70–71
    coordination between community partners and health care organizations during, 18
    possible hazards related to, 2
    response plans for, vii, viii
    security plans for coordination with law enforcement, 71–73
Cleaning organization, strategies for during water contamination emergency, 103–104
CMS. *See* Centers for Medicare & Medicaid Services (CMS)
Coast Guard, U.S., 127
Collaboration and coalition building
    alternative care site arrangements, 17, 22, 34, 52, 156–157, 160
    barriers to, ix
    case study, Bon Secours Baltimore Health System recovery and resilience, 158
    coalition exercises, 137
    community partners, collaboration with, 3, 16–17
    effective emergency management and, 18, 20–21, 31
    emergency manager role in, 4
    health care coalitions, 16–17, 20–21, 63, 137
    importance of, viii–ix
    infectious disease outbreaks management and, 8
    media, coordination and collaboration with, 51
    mutual aid agreements, viii–ix, 21, 34, 137
    preparedness and processes for, 5
    sharing of resources and assets, 59, 63, 64
    vulnerable populations, emergency management of and coalition resources, 119–120
"Communicating Without English in an Emergency Planning Template" (ECHO Minnesota), 45
Communications
    backup communication systems, 38, 52–53
    case study, Yale New Haven Health IT outage, 47–49
    community partners, communication with, 38–39
    contact lists, 38–43, 53, 81
    crisis communications team, 38–39
    crisis standards of care and processes for, 35
    emergency management critical area, viii, xi, xiii, 1–2, 6, 37
    EOP inclusion of procedures for, 38, 43, 53
    external authorities, communication with, 38–39, 44
    first responders, communication strategies for, 121

Government Emergency Telecommunications Service (GETS), 50
hotlines, 46
importance of, 37
law enforcement agencies, communication with, 38, 44, 72
limited English proficiency (LEP) and language barriers, 45
maintenance of emergency equipment, 53
media, communication with, 38–39, 46, 49–50
methods of communication, 38–39, 40, 43
monitoring management processes during exercises, 130
other health care organizations, communication with, 51–52
patients and families, communication with, 38–39, 44–46
preparedness and processes for, 5, 6
privacy and release of information, 40, 46
procedures and processes during emergencies, design of strategy for, 37–38
redundant communication pathways, 6, 53, 79
social media use, 40
staff and licensed independent providers, communication with, 38–43
state and local agencies, communication with, 38–39
suppliers and vendors, communication with, 38–39, 50–51
utilities failures, communication about, 101, 105
Community partners
 alternative care site arrangements, 17, 22, 34, 52, 156–157, 160
 collaboration with, 3, 16–17
 communication with, 38–39
 communitywide exercises with, 130, 133, 134–136
 crisis standards of care and coordination with, 33
 effective emergency management and coordination with, 18, 31
 emergency manager role in coordination of activities with, 4
 health care coalitions, 16–17, 20–21
 HVA development role of, 11–12
 infectious disease outbreaks management and, 8
 organization capabilities, identification of for response and recovery, 16
 sharing of resources and assets, 59, 63, 64
 vulnerable populations, emergency management of and partnerships with, 119–120
Communitywide exercises, 130, 133, 134–136
Computer simulations, 147
Contact lists, 38–43, 53, 81
Contaminated patients. *See also* Decontamination and decontamination facilities

 identification of, staff training on, 77, 88–89
 isolation plans and procedures, 76–77
Continuity of government program, 150
Continuity of operations (COOP)
 activation o plan, 152
 business continuity planning (BCP), 47
 concept of, xii
 downtime and recovery procedures, 79, 106, 149, 152–154, 160
 EOP compared to, 151–152
 EOP integration with, 151–152
 essential functions for recovery, 151
 importance of, 150
 plan and planning for, 79
 planning for and plan development, 150–152, 160
 programs for, 150
 recovery and return to normal operations, 5–6
 utility systems and, 106
Credentialing and privileging
 disaster privileges and volunteer licensed independent practitioners, 79, 94–96
 disaster responsibilities assignment to volunteer practitioners, 79, 94, 96
 primary source verification, 95
 volunteer practitioners, credentialing process for, 80, 86–87, 94–96
Crisis standards of care (CSC), viii, 17, 32–35, 88
Critical access hospitals, xiii
Crowd control, 69, 77
Crozer-Keystone Health System security measures surrounding Pope's visit case study, 14–15
Cultural sensitivity training, 77
Cyber attacks, vii, 2

D

Debriefing sessions for stress management, 85
Decontamination and decontamination facilities
 clean and dirty sides, 75
 exercises to test procedures for, 132
 hazardous materials and waste handling and decontamination plans, 73, 77
 indoor facilities, 74–75, 77
 issues related to, 74–75
 outdoor facilities, 74, 75, 77
 privacy during decontamination, 74, 75
 procedures for, 74–75, 77

staff training for decontamination procedures, 76, 77, 88–90
triage location for patients and decontamination, 113
Disaster Medical Assistance Team (DMAT), 86, 94, 96, 127, 156
Disaster Mortuary Assistance Team (DMORT), 94, 96
Dishwashing, 100
Disruptive behavior, 66
DMAT (Disaster Medical Assistance Team), 86, 94, 96, 127, 156
DMORT (Disaster Mortuary Assistance Team), 94, 96
Downtime and recovery procedures, 47–48, 49, 79, 106, 149, 152–154, 160
Drills. *See* Exercises and drills
Drinking water, 100, 102

E

Earthquake, Kona Community Hospital response to, 126–127
Ebola
    preparedness and response plans for, vi, 8
    staff training on identification and isolation of patients with, 91
    University of Nebraska Medical Center/Nebraska Biocontainment Unit Ebola patients treatment case study, 9, 39, 139–141
ECHO Minnesota, 45
Elderly patients, 60, 62, 63–64, 89, 107, 118–119
Electricity/electrical sources
    alternative sources for, 8, 98
    backup systems, 104–105, 107
    case study, Sutter Medical Center backup power failure, 108–109
    emergency power systems and generators, 98, 99
    EOP and management of during emergencies, 101, 104
    exercises and drills to simulate outages, 101
    failures, planning for, 97
    inspection, testing, and maintenance of, 98, 99
    mitigation activities, 98
    power failure in nursing care centers, 107
    protection of supply, 8
    written contingency plans for management of, 98
Electronic medical records. *See* Medical records/electronic medical records (EMRs)
Elevators, 98, 101
Emergencies and disasters
    accidental disasters, 2
    annual review of planning for, 3
    authority to declare end of emergency, 22
    cessation of services following, 105, 159, 160
    coping strategies following, 86
    decision points in progression of, 111–112
    definition of disaster, 1
    definition of emergency, 1
    evaluation of actual responses to or exercises, 133, 137, 141–142, 143–146, 147
    intentional events, 2
    multiple emergency situations, 2, 9, 112, 132
    natural disasters, 2
    possible hazards related to, vii, 1, 2
    responses to, review of by leadership, 3
    reunification of patients and family members, 126
Emergency department (ED)
    entrances, monitoring of, 66
    first responder awareness training for staff in, 89
    plans and procedures for surge of incoming patients, 112–114
    space management in, 62–63
Emergency management
    all-hazards approach to, xii, 1, 8
    best practices for success, 18, 20–24
    collaboration and coalition building for, viii–ix
    critical areas of, viii, xi, xiii, 1–2, 3, 6, 8 (*see also* specific areas)
    critical areas of, monitoring management of during exercises, 130
    definition of, 1
    effective emergency management, xi, 18, 20–24, 31
    importance of, vii
    individual responsible for, 3–4
    leadership role in, xi, xii, 3–4, 8
    performance improvement decisions, 142
    standards on, xii
    strong and flexible emergency planning, 9
    team approach to planning for, 4
Emergency Management (EM) standards
    chapter for in accreditation manuals, vii, xiii
    communications during emergencies (EM.02.02.01), 37
    disaster privileges and volunteer licensed independent practitioners (EM.02.02.13), 79, 96
    disaster responsibilities assignment to volunteer practitioners (EM.02.02.15), 79, 94, 96
    emergency management planning, evaluation of effectiveness of (EM.03.01.01), 129
Emergency Operations Plan (EOP)

evaluation of effectiveness of (EM.03.01.03), 129
planning activities prior to development of
(EM.01.01.01), 1, 9
requirement for (EM.02.01.01), 1, 9, 37, 55, 65, 79, 97,
111, 129, 149
HICS and compliance with, 25
importance and urgency of, vii
NIMS and compliance with, 25
patients, management of during emergencies
(EM.02.02.11), 111
resources and assets, management of during emergencies
(EM.02.02.03), 55
safety and security, management of during emergencies
(EM.02.02.05), 65
staff, management of during emergencies
(EM.02.02.07), 79
staff training requirements, 59
utilities, management of during emergencies
(EM.02.02.09), 97
Emergency Management, Office of, 87
Emergency management phases, 3, 4–6. *See also* Mitigation;
Preparedness; Recovery; Response
Emergency Management Plan (EMP), xv, 3
Emergency managers
appointment of by leadership, 3–4, 8
health care coalitions role of, 21
responsibilities of, 3–4, 8
Emergency Medical Treatment and Active Labor Act, 34
Emergency Operations Plan (EOP)
all-hazards EOP, 15–18
authority to initiate and terminate phases of, 16
chemical, biological, and radioactive materials, safety and
security threats from, 68
communications procedures in, 38, 43, 53
COOP compared to, 151–152
COOP integration with, 151–152
evaluation of exercises or actual responses, 133, 137,
141–142, 143–146, 147
function and purpose of, 2–3, 9, 15–18
home care, management of critical areas for, 60
HVA and development of, 3, 8, 10–13, 15, 31
importance of, 9
initiation of, notification of staff of, 38
initiation of in preparation for an emergency, xi
leadership role in development of, 3
modifications to, 133, 142, 147
preparedness and capabilities to implement, 5
requirement for, vii, 31

requirement for (EM.02.01.01), 1, 9, 37, 55, 65, 79, 97,
111, 129, 149
supplies, management of availability of, 60–61
testing and evaluation of, 129–133, 137–138,
141–142, 147
training and education activities outline as part of, 87
utilities management procedures in, 101, 104
Emory University, 141
Environmental Protection Agency (EPA), 73, 76
Environment of Care (EC) standard on hazardous materials
and waste management, 73
Environment of care case study, Carilion Franklin Memorial
Hospital staff training, 82–83
Equipment
decontamination, access to equipment for, 74, 75
maintenance of emergency equipment, 53
mitigation activities, 98
organization capabilities, identification of for response and
recovery, 16
recovery after damage from emergencies and disasters, 156
Escalating events
decision points in progression of, 112
exercises to evaluation policies and procedures for, 35,
132, 147
patient safety and provision of care during, 2–3
Evacuations and evacuation procedures
alternative care sites, 17, 22, 62, 115
authority to declare end of emergency and return of
evacuated patients, 22
case studies
Beth Israel Deaconess Medical Center
communitywide exercise and operating room
evacuation drill, 134–136
Kona Community Hospital earthquake response,
126–127
Mercy Hospital Joplin tornado event and evacuation,
92–93
decision points in progression of emergencies, 114–115
development of evacuation plans, viii, 22
drills to test procedures, 5, 115
long term care settings, plans for patients in, 62, 118–119
patient safety during evacuations, 63–64
plans and procedures for, 115
power failure in nursing care centers decisions about, 107
resources, equipment, and staff for, 63–64
staff training for, 94
timing of evacuation orders, 22
transportation arrangements for, 60, 62, 64, 115

utility failures and decisions about, 105, 107, 109
vulnerable populations, decisions about, 62, 107, 115
Exercises and drills
   active shooter incidents, 69
   after-action debriefings, 137, 143–146, 147
   bomb threat drills, 73
   case studies
      Beth Israel Deaconess Medical Center community-wide exercise and operating room evacuation drill, 134–136
      Carilion Franklin Memorial Hospital staff training, 82–83
      Mercy Hospital Joplin tornado event and evacuation, 92–93
      University of Nebraska Medical Center/Nebraska Biocontainment Unit Ebola patients treatment, drilling and model development for, 139–141
   coalition exercises, 137
   crisis standards of care, drills and simulations to identify deficiencies, 35
   design of, 147
   emergency management critical area, monitoring management processes during exercises, 130
   environment of care drills, 82–83
   escalating events, exercises to evaluation policies and procedures for, 35, 132, 147
   evacuation procedures, drills to test, 5, 115
   evaluation of exercises or actual responses, 133, 137, 141–142, 143–146, 147
   frequency of, 129, 130
   goals of, 131
   health care coalitions and participation in, 16–17, 21
   law enforcement agencies, cooperative drills with, 72–73
   monitoring response to, 133, 137, 142
   multiple emergency situations, exercises to test response to, 132
   National Disaster Medical System exercise, viii
   patient placement exercise, viii
   personnel safety in laboratories, 68
   planning for, 130–133, 138
   preparedness, exercises to identify gaps in, 5
   requirement for, 35
   respiratory emergency scenario and ventilator-use proficiency, 59
   shelter-in-place procedures, exercises on, 90, 94
   stand-alone response, exercise to test, 132
   surge events, exercises to evaluation policies and procedures for, 35

   training and education of staff, vii
   types of, 130–131
   utility outages, 101
Explosive events. *See* Chemical, biological, radiological, nuclear, explosive (CBRNE) events
External authorities, communication with, 38–39, 44

F

FAA (Federal Aviation Administration), 137
Facilities, recovery after damage from emergencies and disasters, 156
Federal Aviation Administration (FAA), 137
Federal Emergency Management Agency (FEMA), 7, 44, 151, 154
FEMA (Federal Emergency Management Agency), 7, 44, 151, 154
Fires
   facilities, recovery after damage from, 156
   HVA sample, 13
   possible hazards related to, 2
   response plans for, xi
Flooding incidents
   case study, Sutter Medical Center backup power failure, 108–109
   facilities, recovery after damage from, 156
   HVA sample, 13
   possible hazards related to, 1, 2
   response plans for, viii, xi
Food
   exercises to test emergency procedures for, 132
   management of and obtaining and replenishing supply of, 61–62
   mitigation activities and alternative supply chain for, 5
   water contamination emergencies and preparation of, 100, 102
Forensic patients, 73
France, terrorist attack in, 72
Francis, Pope, 14–15
Freeman Health System, 93
Fuel
   alternative sources for, 8
   backup systems, 104–105
   exercises and drills to simulate outages, 101
   management of and obtaining and replenishing supply of, 61–62
   mitigation activities and alternative supply chain for, 5

protection of supply, 8
transportation assistance for patients during emergencies and priority access to, 60
written contingency plans for management of, 98
Functional exercises, 130

G

Gap analysis, 11, 12, 99
Geriatric patients, 60, 62, 63–64, 89, 107, 118–119
GETS (Government Emergency Telecommunications Service), 50
Glossary, 161–164
Government and federal agencies. *See also* specific department and agencies
coordination with, 71–73
disaster response teams, 86
Government Emergency Telecommunications Service (GETS), 50
hazardous materials and waste, standards and recommendations for safe handling of, 73, 76
instructors for staff training from, 87
Gray, Freddie, 18, 70
Grief counseling, 79, 83, 86, 122

H

Hand washing and hygiene, 89, 100–101, 102, 115
Hawaii Health System Corporation, 127
Hazardous materials and waste
chemical, biological, and radioactive materials in laboratories, safety and security threats from, 68
containment of pathogens and toxins, 68
decontamination, handling and disposal of waste from, 74, 75, 77
HAZMAT (hazardous materials) events, 2
management of, 72, 73, 76, 77
security precautions for, 72
staff training for management of, 89–90
storage of supplies and agents in, 68
types of, 73
Hazardous Waste Operations and Emergency Response (HAZWOPER) standard (OSHA), 88–90
Hazard vulnerability analysis (HVA)
EOP development role of, 3, 8, 10–13, 15, 31
evaluation and updating of, 3, 11–12, 147
function and purpose of, 3, 10
identification of hazards, 10, 31, 151–152
leadership role in development of, 3
mitigation activities based on, 5, 10, 15
multiple HVAs for larger systems, 10
preparedness planning based on, 10
prioritizing hazards/risks, 3, 10–13, 31
process for development of, 3, 10, 11
recovery planning based on, 10
response planning based on, 10
sample planning tool, 11, 13
supplies, HVA to identify needs and adequate supply levels, 55–56, 59, 61
Health and Human Services, U.S. Department of (HHS)
Assistant Secretary for Preparedness and Response (ASPR), 7, 87, 90, 141
crisis standards of care development, 32–35
Ebola treatment and best practices development, 141
Technical Resources, Assistance Center, and Information Exchange (TRACIE), 20
ventilators from SNS, 59
Health care coalitions, 16–17, 20–21, 63, 137
Health conditions, release of information about, 40, 46
Health First–Cape Canaveral Hospital hurricane events and and recovery case study, 155–156
Health First–Palm Bay Hospital active shooter incident case study, 67
Health Insurance Portability and Accountability Act (HIPAA), 34, 46
Heating, ventilating, and air-conditioning (HVAC) systems, 98, 104
Helipads, 69
HICS (Hospital Incident Command System), 22, 25, 83
Highland Clarksburg Hospital snow storm event case study, 19–20
Hilo Medical Center, 127
HIPAA (Health Insurance Portability and Accountability Act), 34, 46
Home care organizations
Emergency Management (EM) standards for, xiii
emergency management for patients in, 62
EOP and management of critical areas for, 60
transportation assistance for patients during emergencies, 60
Homeland Security, U.S. Department of
Government Emergency Telecommunications Service (GETS), 50

limited English proficiency (LEP) patients and families, communication with, 45
Hope is not a strategy, xi
Hospice settings, emergency management for patients in, 62
Hospital Incident Command System (HICS), 22, 25, 83
Hotlines, 46
Hudson Valley MACE (Mutual Aid Coordinating Entity), viii
Hurricanes
    case study, Cape Canaveral Hospital hurricane events and and recovery, 155–156
    health care coalitions and response to, 17
    HVA sample, 13
    mutual aid and assistance in response to damage from, viii
Hygiene and hand washing, 89, 100–101, 102, 115

I

Ice storms, viii
Illinois Emergency Management Agency (IEMA), 76, 154
Incident command structure (ICS)
    authority to initiate and terminate EOP phases, identification of, 16
    communication with external authorities through, 44
    concept and function of, 22, 31
    crisis management with, vii
    EOP implementation and response activities, 5
    EOP requirement for, 16
    framework for, 22, 25
    functional areas of, 22, 24
    importance of, 16
    leadership responsibilities, 22, 24
    leadership support for, 3
    requirement for, 22
    responsibilities of incident commander, 22, 26–30
    staff responsibilities, definition/clarification of through, 16, 22, 24, 84–85
Incident command structure, community
    integration of organization into, 22, 24
    National Incident Management System (NIMS), 7, 24, 25
    organization role in, leadership decisions about, 3
Industrial accidents
    possible hazards related to, 2
    preparedness and response plans for, xii, 9
Infant abductions, 5, 72–73

Infection Control and Prevention (IC) standard on staff training requirements, 59
Infection control/isolation
    staff training for, 90, 91
    syndromic surveillance, 90
Infectious disease outbreaks
    case study
        University of Nebraska Medical Center/Nebraska Biocontainment Unit Ebola patients treatment, 9, 39
        University of Nebraska Medical Center/Nebraska Biocontainment Unit Ebola patients treatment, drilling and model development for, 139–141
    expertise of medical staff in planning procedures for, 8
    health care coalitions and response to, 17
    medications for, obtaining and replenishing supply of, 57
    possible hazards related to, 1, 2
    preparedness and capabilities to manage, 5
    preparedness and response plans for, vii, viii, xi, xii, 8
    staff training on control/isolation precautions, 90, 91
    syndromic surveillance, 90
    triage location for patients, 113
Influenza
    flu vaccine availability, 21
    medications for outbreaks, obtaining and replenishing supply of, 57
    pandemic flu, preparedness and response to, 5
    supply shortages during outbreaks of, 21
Information Management (IM) standard on continuity of information management processes (IM.01.01.03), 149
Information technology (IT)
    advancements in and security of information, xii
    case study, Yale New Haven Health IT outage, 47–49
    downtime and recovery procedures, 47–48, 49, 79, 152–154
    mitigation activities for, 5
    vulnerabilities in disaster response, xii
Information technology disaster recovery (IT DR) program, 150–152, 154
Institute of Medicine, 32
Internal security, 65–71
Interpretation and translation services, 45, 119
Isolation plans and procedures, 76–77, 90, 132
"I Speak" posters, 45

J

The Joint Commission
    cessation of services, notification about, 105, 160
    Emergency Management Portal, 7
Jonas, Winter Storm, xi

K

Key to chapter features, xiv
Kona Community Hospital earthquake response case study, 126–127

L

Laboratories
    access control and authorized access, 68
    chemical, biological, and radioactive materials in, safety and security threats from, 68
    containment of pathogens and toxins, 68
    Emergency Management (EM) standards for, xiii
    personnel safety and training of staff, 68
    safe handling of specimens, procedures for, 68
    storage of supplies and agents in, 68
Language barriers and communication with vulnerable populations, 45
Larsen, Erik, viii
Law enforcement agencies
    access to facilities by, 67, 69
    active shooter incidents, response to, 67, 69
    coalition exercises, 137
    communication with, 38, 44, 72
    coordination with, 12, 18, 31, 67, 69, 71–73, 77
    evacuations and transportation arrangements coordination with, 60, 64
    exercises and drills with, 72–73
    Government Emergency Telecommunications Service (GETS), 50
    hazards identification and coordination with, 10
    hospital plans and life safety drawings, access to, 67, 69
    instructors for staff training from, 87
    privacy and release of information during emergencies, 40
Laws and regulations
    CMS regulation and policy updates, 7
    crisis standards of care, legal issues related to, 34
    emergency preparedness and response laws and regulations, 7
    state and local laws and regulations, 7
Leadership
    coping strategies following disasters, 86
    emergency management and preparedness role of, xi, xii, 3–4, 8
    evaluation of exercises and actual responses to emergencies, 142
    HVA development role of, 3
    ICS responsibilities of, 22, 24
    ICS support from, 3
    risk management role of, 3
Leadership (LD) standards
    effective management of programs, services, sites, or departments (LD.04.01.05), 1, 9
    performance improvement priorities (LD.04.04.01), 1, 9, 129, 142
Licensed independent practitioners
    communication with, 38–43
    disaster privileges and volunteer licensed independent practitioners, 79
    emergency response role of, 85
    integration of into training activities, 85
    volunteer practitioners, credentialing process for, 80, 86–87
Limited English proficiency (LEP) patients and families, 45, 89, 119
Local agencies. *See* State and local agencies

M

MACE (Mutual Aid Coordinating Entity), viii–ix, 21, 137
Massachusetts General Hospital, 134
Mass-casualty incidents
    exercises to test procedures for, 131–132
    grief counseling or pastoral counseling following, 79, 83, 122
    health care coalitions and response to, 17
    possible hazards related to, 1, 2
    preparedness and response plans for, viii, 9
Media
    communication with, 38–39, 46, 49–50
    coordination and collaboration with, 51
Medical gas and vacuum systems, 98, 101
Medical records/electronic medical records (EMRs)
    case studies
        Mercy Hospital Joplin tornado event and evacuation, 93

Yale New Haven Health IT outage, 47–49
documenting and tracking clinical information, 120–125, 128
sample patient tracking forms, 123–125
technology advancements in and security of electronic records, xii
Medical Reserve Corps (MRC), 94, 96
Medications
civil unrest incidents and availability of, 18
long term care settings, plans for patients in, 62
management of and sources for, 57
Mental Health America (National Mental Health Association), 86
Mercy Health 96-hour operational capabilities chart, 22, 23
Mercy Hospital Joplin tornado event and evacuation case study, 92–93
Minnesota Department of Health and ECHO Minnesota, 45
Mitigation
activities for, 4–5, 15
alternative supply chain identification, 5, 21
emergency manager role in, 4
EOP role in, 3
HVA and activities for, 5, 10, 15
leadership role in decisions about, 3
medication resource management, 57
utility systems, 5, 98, 106, 109
workplace violence safety and security concerns example, 12
Mortuary services, 120
MRC (Medical Reserve Corps), 94, 96
Mutual aid agreements, viii–ix, 34, 137
Mutual Aid Coordinating Entity (MACE), viii–ix, 21, 137

N

National Disaster Medical System (NDMS) exercise, 137
National Disaster Medical System exercise, viii
National Ebola Training and Education Center, 141
National Fire Protection Association (NFPA), 7
disaster/emergency management code, 7
health care facilities code, 7
National Incident Management System (NIMS), 7, 24, 25
National Mental Health Association (Mental Health America), 86
National Resource Center on Advancing Emergency Preparedness for Culturally Diverse Communities, 45
National Response Framework (NRF), 7
NDMS (National Disaster Medical System) exercise, 137

NFPA (National Fire Protection Association), 7
NIMS (National Incident Management System), 7, 24, 25
96-hour operational capabilities, 17, 21–22, 23
NRF (National Response Framework), 7
Nuclear events. See Chemical, biological, radiological, nuclear, explosive (CBRNE) events
Nuclear Regulatory Commission (NRC), 76
Nursing care centers
communications procedures for, 43
emergency management for patients in, 62, 118–119
management of resources and supplies after September 11 attacks, 57
population-specific training for staff, 89
power failure in, 107

O

Occupational Health and Safety Administration (OSHA)
First Receiver guidelines, staff training on, 77, 88–90
first responder awareness training, 89
hazardous materials and waste, standards and recommendations for safe handling of, 76
Hazardous Waste Operations and Emergency Response (HAZWOPER) standard, 88–90
information from and access to information, 7
instructors for staff training from, 87
staff training on safety protection policies, 88
water contamination emergencies, recommendations during, 100–101
OSHA. See Occupational Health and Safety Administration (OSHA)

P

Palliative care, 35
Pastoral counseling and spiritual resources, 43, 46, 79, 83, 86, 122
Patient care and clinical and support activities
alternative care sites, 17, 22, 34, 52, 62, 127, 156–157, 160
case study, Kona Community Hospital earthquake response, 126–127
crisis standards of care, viii, 17, 32–35, 88
decision points in progression of emergencies, 111–112
disparities in services, mitigation of risks of, 119–120
documenting and tracking clinical information, 120–125, 128

emergency management critical area, viii, xi, xiii, 1–2, 8, 111
mental health needs and counseling, 43, 46, 115, 120, 122
monitoring management processes during exercises, 130
96-hour operational capabilities, 17, 21–22, 23
recovery and return to normal operations, 5–6, 149–150, 160
sanitation and hygiene facilities, 115
surge of incoming patients, 112–114
vulnerable populations, 118–120, 128
Patients, use of terminology, xv
Patients and families
    communication with, 38–39, 44–46
    limited English proficiency (LEP) patients and families, communication with, 45, 89, 119
    privacy and release of information during emergencies, 40, 46
    reunification of patients and family members, 126
Payroll operations and backup compensation plans, 79, 157
Pediatric population, 5, 60, 72–73, 89, 118
Personal protective equipment (PPE), 17, 21, 50, 59, 61, 75, 89
Police. *See* Law enforcement agencies
Preparedness
    budget and financial plan development, 56, 154
    capabilities and activities for, 4–5
    case study, Crozer-Keystone Health System security measures surrounding Pope's visit, 14–15
    collaboration with community for preparedness planning, 16–17
    commitment to organizationwide, 8
    emergency manager role in, 4
    EOP implementation and, 5
    EOP role in, 3
    expertise of medical staff in planning procedures, 8
    health care coalitions and planning for, 16–17, 20–21
    laws and regulations resources, 7
    leadership role in decisions about, 3
    medication resource management, 57
    ongoing activities for, 8
    resources and assets for, 3
    team approach to, 4
    utility systems, 101, 106
    workplace violence safety and security concerns example, 12
Press office and public information officer (PIO), 38, 46, 49–50
Prison inmates, 73
Privacy and release of information during emergencies, 40, 46

Public health emergencies (PHEs), ventilators from SNS for, 58–59
Public information officer (PIO), 38, 46, 49–50

R

Radiological events. *See* Chemical, biological, radiological, nuclear, explosive (CBRNE) events
Radiological Task Force (RTF), 76
    Radiological Assessment Field Team (RAFT), 76
    Radiological Emergency Assessment Center (REAC), 76
Recovery. *See also* Continuity of operations (COOP)
    activities and strategies for, 4–6, 18, 149–154, 156–157, 159
    after-action review, 154
    alternative care sites and, 156–157, 160
    authority to declare end of emergency and return of evacuated patients, 22
    authority to initiate and terminate EOP phase for, 16
    case studies
    Bon Secours Baltimore Health System recovery and resilience, 158
    Cape Canaveral Hospital hurricane events and and recovery, 155–156
    downtime and recovery procedures, 47–48, 49, 79, 106, 149, 152–154, 160
    emergency manager role in, 4
    EOP role in, 3
    essential functions for, 151
    finances and funding for recovery activities, 154
    health care coalitions and resilience of, 16–17, 20–21
    leadership role in planning for, 3
    normal operations, restoring, 149–150, 160
    organization capabilities, identification of for response and recovery, 16
    patient safety and, 5–6
    priorities for, 149
    successful recovery, 149
    utility systems, 106, 107
    workplace violence safety and security concerns example, 12
Red Cross, 76
Resources and assets. *See also* Supplies/medical supplies
    alternative sources for, 5, 17
    assignment of resources for preparedness activities, 3
    budget and financial plan for obtaining and replenishing resources, 56, 154

case studies
   Highland Clarksburg Hospital snow storm event, 19–20
   St. Margaret's Home and September 11 attacks, 57
   University of Maryland Medical Center snow storm event, 19–20
community collaboration and sharing of, 59, 63, 64
emergency management critical area, viii, xiii, 1–2, 6, 55
health care coalitions and sharing of during disasters, 16–17, 20–21
HVA to identify needs and adequate supply levels, 55–56
management of, xii
mitigation activities and alternative supply chain for, 5
monitoring and management of, requirement for, 17
monitoring management processes during exercises, 130
96-hour operational capabilities, 17, 21–22, 23
space management, 62–63, 64
Respirators, 21, 59, 61, 75
Response
   activities and procedures for, 4–5, 15–16
   authority to initiate and terminate EOP phase for, 16
   emergency manager role in, 4
   EOP implementation and, 5
   EOP role in, 3
   health care coalitions and resilience of, 16–17, 20–21
   laws and regulations resources, 7
   organization capabilities, identification of for response and recovery, 16
   patient safety and, 5
   utility systems, 106
   workplace violence safety and security concerns example, 12
Response plans
   active shooter incidents, vii, viii, xii, 8, 69
   development of, vii, viii
   preparedness and testing of, 5
Riots. *See* Civil unrest incidents
Risk management. *See also* Hazard vulnerabilty analysis (HVA)
   leadership role in, 3
   prioritizing hazards/risks, 3, 4, 10–13, 31
   risk-identification training for staff, 88

S

Safety and security of staff, patients, and visitors. *See also* Active shooter incidents
   access control and authorized access, 66–69
   case studies

      Crozer-Keystone Health System security measures surrounding Pope's visit, 14–15
      University of Maryland Medical Center continuity of operations during civil unrest and riots, 70–71
   crowd control, 69, 77
   decontamination and decontamination facilities, 74–75, 76, 77
   disruptive behavior and, 66
   emergency management critical area, viii, xi, xiii, 1–2, 6, 65
   employee screening, 68
   entrances, monitoring of, 66
   evacuations, patient safety during, 63–64
   forensic patients, difficulties associated with, 73
   hazardous materials and waste, management of, 73, 76, 77
   infant abductions, elimination of opportunities for, 5
   inside threats, 71
   internal security, 65–71
   isolation plans and procedures, 76–77
   law enforcement agencies, coordination with, 71–73, 77
   limited access to specific areas, 66
   mitigation activities for, 5
   monitoring management processes during exercises, 130
   reference materials for staff, 81
   response activities and, 5
   safety failures, 65
   scalability of security plans, 71–72
   security failures, 65
   staff training on safety protection policies, 88
St. Margaret's Home, 57
Sandy, Superstorm, viii, 122
Sanitation and hygiene facilities, 115
September 11 attacks
   emergency preparedness responsibilities following, vii
   St. Margaret's Home resources and supplies management following, 57
Shelter in place
   long term care settings, plans for patients in, 62, 118–119
   power failure in nursing care centers decisions about, 107
   staff training and drilling on procedures, 90, 94
Simulations, 130, 147
Social media, 40
Space management, 62–63, 64
Specimens, procedures for safe handling of, 68
Spiritual resources and pastoral counseling, 43, 46, 79, 83, 86, 122
Staff. *See also* Training, education, and orientation of staff; Workplace violence
   communication with, 38–43, 81

coping strategies and counseling for after disasters, 79, 83, 86, 122
employee screening and security threats, 68
expertise of medical staff in preparedness activities, 8
health care coalitions and manpower pool for disasters, 16–17
identification of during emergencies, 66, 94
multilingual staff and communication with LEP patients and families, 45
payroll operations and backup compensation plans, 79, 157
physical needs of, planning for, 81, 83
preparedness and capabilities of, 5
role and responsibilities
    assignment of and staff understanding of, 80
    critical areas of response, 83–84
    emergency management, role in, vii
    emergency management critical area, viii, xi, xiii, 1–2, 6, 8, 79
    ICS and definition/clarification of, 16, 22, 24, 84–85
    monitoring management processes during exercises, 130
    shifting of during emergencies, 79, 83–84
    training for (*see* Training, education, and orientation of staff)
safety reference materials for, 81
stress, strategies and support for management of, 83, 85
support for during emergencies, 79, 81, 83
transportation for, 81
Staffing
    adequate levels of, 80, 84
    case studies
        Highland Clarksburg Hospital snow storm event, 19–20
        University of Maryland Medical Center snow storm event, 19–20
    emergency conditions, staffing plan for, 81
    normal operations, staffing for return to, 157
    strategies for during events, 84, 157
State and local agencies
    communication with, 38–39
    communitywide exercises, 130, 133, 134–136
    coordination with, 71–73
    crisis standards of care, legal issues related to, 34
    disaster response teams, 86
    effective emergency management and coordination with, 18, 31
    health care coalitions, 16–17, 20–21
    instructors for staff training from, 87
    radiological and nuclear events, response to, 76
    state and local laws and regulations, 7

Sterilization processes, 98
Stewart Air National Guard Base, 137
Strategic National Stockpile (SNS), 57, 58–59
Stress, strategies and support for staff to manage, 83, 85
Supplies/medical supplies
    alternative supply chain for, 5, 21, 63
    common supplies needed in emergency situations, 61
    communication with suppliers and vendors, 38–39, 50–51
    decontamination, access to supplies for, 74, 75
    EOP and management of availability of, 60–61
    evacuations, resources and equipment for, 63–64
    exercises to test emergency procedures for, 132
    HVA to identify needs and adequate supply levels, 55–56, 59, 61
    management of and caches of emergency medical supplies, 59–61, 64
    96-hour operational capabilities, 17, 21–22, 23
    nonmedical supplies, 61–62
    obtaining and replenishing, 55–56, 63
    preparedness and relationship with suppliers, 21, 63, 64
    preparedness and supply chain for, 5
    sharing of with coalition partners, 63, 64
Surge events
    definition of, 1
    exercises to evaluation policies and procedures for, 35
    exercises to test procedures for, 131–132
    plans and procedures for surge of incoming patients, 112–114
    preparedness and capabilities to manage, 5, 9
    space management during, 62–63
Sutter Medical Center backup power failure case study, 108–109
Syndromic surveillance, 90
Systems and processes
    crisis standards of care and, 35
    management of, xii

T

Tabletop exercises, 130, 147
Teams and teamwork
    crisis communications team, 38–39
    for emergency management planning, 4
    exercises to promote, 5
    infectious disease outbreaks management and, 8
Technical Resources, Assistance Center, and Information Exchange (TRACIE), 20

Terrorist attacks
    possible hazards related to, 1, 2
    response plans for, xi, xii
    security plans for coordination with law enforcement agencies, 71–73

Training, education, and orientation of staff
    active shooter incidents, 69, 88
    case studies
        Carilion Franklin Memorial Hospital staff training, 82–83
        Mercy Hospital Joplin tornado event and evacuation, 92–93
    CBRNE events, 88
    crisis standards of care, orientation on, 33
    cultural sensitivity training, 77
    decontamination procedures, 76, 77, 88–90
    effective emergency management and, xi
    emergency response role, training for, 80–81, 87–94, 96
    environment of care orientation and training, 82–83
    EOP, orientation to, 80
    EOP outline of training and education activities, 87
    evacuations and evacuation procedures, 94
    exercises for, vii
    first responders, training of, 89, 121
    formats of, 87
    frequency of sessions, 87, 90
    health care coalitions and participation in, 16–17
    instructors for, in-house and external, 87
    personnel safety in laboratories, 68
    population-specific training, 89, 96, 118–120
    population-specific training for staff, 96
    preparedness and capabilities of staff, 5
    requirement for, 87
    risk-identification training, 88
    safety protection policies, 88
    shelter-in-place procedures and training, 90, 94
    standards on, vii
    topics for, 87, 88–91, 94
    train-the-trainer presentations, 59
    treatment under adverse conditions, 90
    triage procedures, 87, 88
    ventilators from SNS, training personnel on use of, 58–59
    water contamination, training in identifying and treating, 97

Translation and interpretation services, 45, 119

Transportation
    arrangements and assistance for patients during emergencies, 60, 62, 64, 115
    case study, Kona Community Hospital earthquake response, 127
    home care settings, plans for patients in, 60
    long term care settings, plans for patients in, 62, 118–119
    safety and security and control of vehicular access, 66, 68–69
    for staff, 81

Transportation accidents, 1, 2

Triage
    case study, Mercy Hospital Joplin tornado event and evacuation, 92–93
    color-coded tag system, 114
    crisis standards of care and processes for, 35, 88
    exercises to test procedures for, 132
    patient placement exercise, viii
    plans and procedures for, 112–114
    preparedness and testing of plan for, 5
    sample triage form, 113, 116–117
    staff training for, 87, 88

U

University of Maryland Medical Center continuity of operations during civil unrest and riots case study, 70–71

University of Maryland Medical Center snow storm event case study, 19–20

University of Nebraska Medical Center/Nebraska Biocontainment Unit Ebola patients treatment case study, 9, 39, 139–141

Urban Shield exercise, 134–136

Utilities
    alternative sources for, 8, 98
    backup systems, 104–105, 107
    case study, Sutter Medical Center backup power failure, 108–109
    downtime and recovery procedures, 106, 152–154
    emergency management critical area, viii, xiii, 1–2, 8, 97
    EOP and management of during emergencies, 101, 104
    exercises and drills to simulate outages, 101
    external emergencies, 97
    failure of, communication about, 101, 105
    failures, planning for, 97–101, 109
    internal sabotage and intentional damage, 97
    management of during emergencies, xii, 101–105, 107, 109
    mitigation activities for, 5, 98, 106, 109
    monitoring management processes during exercises, 130

possible hazards related to failure of, 2
preparedness activities, 101
preparedness activities for, 106
recovery after failures, 106, 107
recovery and damage from emergencies and disasters, 156
response to failures, 106
written contingency plans for management of, 98

V

Ventilators from Strategic National Stockpile (SNS), 58–59
Volunteer staff/practitioners, 95
    credentialing process for licensed independent practitioners, 80, 86–87, 94–95
    decisions to use, 86
    disaster privileges and volunteer licensed independent practitioners, 79, 94–96
    disaster responsibilities assignment to volunteer practitioners, 79, 94, 96
    licensed volunteers, 86–87, 95–96
    sources of, 86, 94–95
    training of, 86
Vulnerable populations
    evacuation decisions, 62, 107, 115
    forensic patients, 73
    health care coalitions and identification and planning for needs of, 17
    limited English proficiency (LEP) patients and families, communication with, 45, 119
    long term care settings, plans for patients in, 62, 118–119
    patient care during emergencies and disasters, 118–120, 128
    population-specific training for staff, 89, 96, 118–120
    power failure in nursing care centers, 107
    shelter-in-place procedures and training, 94, 118–119

W

Water
    alternative sources for, 5, 8, 98, 104
    backup systems, 104–105
    boil water notices, 100–101, 102–103
    contaminated water supply
        advisories, notifications, and warnings about, 102–103
        cleaning organization, strategies for, 103–104
        communication about, 103
        management of risks associated with, 102–104
        precautions during contamination emergencies, 100–101
        response to, 103–104
        staff training in identifying and treating, 97
        types of contaminants, 102
    contingency plans for management of, 98, 104
    decontamination, disposal of water used for, 74, 75, 77
    EOP and management of during emergencies, 101, 104
    exercises and drills to simulate outages, 101
    management of and obtaining and replenishing supply of, 61–62
    mitigation activities for, 5, 98
    OSHA standards on, 100–101
    protection of supply, 8
    system failures, planning for, 97, 104
Weather occurences. *See also* Hurricanes
    case studies
        Cape Canaveral Hospital hurricane events and and recovery, 155–156
        Highland Clarksburg Hospital snow storm event, 19–20
        Mercy Hospital Joplin tornado event and evacuation, 92–93
        University of Maryland Medical Center snow storm event, 19–20
    decision points in progression of, 112
    health care coalitions and response to, 17
    HVA sample, 13
    ice storms, viii
    possible hazards related to, 1, 2
    response plans for incidents related to, viii, xii
    Winter Storm Jonas, preparedness for and response to, xi
Web-based applications for communication, 40
Wen, Leana S., 18
Westchester County Airport, 137
Westchester County Department of Health, viii
White Plains
    coalition building and the emergency preparedness task force, viii–ix
    exercises and training for emergencies, ix
    White Plains Fire Department, viii, ix
    White Plains Police Department, viii, ix
White Plains Hospital
    emergency preparedness plans and exercises, development of, viii
    evacuation plans development, viii

Wireless Priority Service (WPS) program, 50

Workplace violence
    safety and security and threat from, 71
    safety and security concerns example, 12
    staff training to recognize behaviors and read indicators
        of threat, 71

Y

Yale New Haven Health IT outage case study, 47–49